Drug-Related Problems in the Elderly

Patrik Midlöv · Tommy Eriksson · Annika Kragh

Drug-Related Problems in the Elderly

Springer

Dr. Patrik Midlöv
Lund University
Faculty of Medicine
SE-221 00 Lund
Sweden
Patrik.Midlov@skane.se
patrik.midlov@med.lu.se

Dr. Tommy Eriksson
Apoteket Farmaci AB
and
Lund University
Faculty of Medicine
SE-221 00 Lund
Sweden
tommy.eriksson@apoteketfarmaci.se

Dr. Annika Kragh
Lund University
Faculty of Medicine
SE-221 00 Lund
Sweden
annika.kraghekstam@skane.se

ISBN 978-90-481-2445-9 e-ISBN 978-90-481-2446-6
DOI 10.1007/978-90-481-2446-6
Springer Dordrecht Heidelberg London New York

Library of Congress Control Number: 2009926974

Printed on acid-free paper

Springer is part of Springer Science+Business Media (www.springer.com)

Preface

Drug-related problems in the elderly is intended to serve as a source of information and clinical support in geriatric pharmacotherapy for students as well as all health care professionals, e.g. physicians, nurses and pharmacists. Pharmacotherapy is of great importance to all mankind. Drugs are however powerful and must be handled appropriately. This is especially important for elderly patients.

Drug-related problem is not a major subject in most university programmes in medicine or pharmacy. When there is no specific course, there is often no book covering the topic. In our view, as teachers at various university courses, there has been a shortage of literature that reflects the most important aspects of drug-related problems in the elderly. Medical practitioners, nurses and pharmacists, need to have this knowledge to be able to serve their patients in the best way.

This book covers most aspects of drug-related problems in the elderly. With better knowledge of drug-related difficulties and risks we hope that elderly will have fewer drug-related problems and benefit more from their pharmacotherapy.

Lund, Sweden Patrik Midlöv
Lund, Sweden Tommy Eriksson
Lund, Sweden Annika Kragh

Contents

1 Aging and Drugs 1
1.1 Introduction 1
1.2 Epidemiology 2
1.3 Drug Related Problems 2
1.4 Evidence Based Medicine 3
1.5 Polypharmacy 4
1.6 General Improved Quality 4
1.7 Specific Problems, Consequences, and Improvements 5
1.8 Conclusions 6
References 6

2 Physiological Alterations with Aging 9
2.1 Introduction 9
2.2 Pharmacokinetics 10
2.2.1 Absorption of Drugs 10
2.2.2 Distribution of Drugs 10
2.2.3 Metabolism 12
2.2.4 Renal Elimination 12
2.2.5 Water and Electrolyte Balance 13
2.3 Pharmacodynamics 14
2.3.1 Cardiovascular Effects 14
2.3.2 Central Nervous System 15
2.4 Drug-Drug Interactions 15
2.5 Drug-Disease Interactions 16
2.6 Adverse Drug Reactions 16
2.7 Adverse Drug Withdrawal Events 17
2.8 Conclusions 17
References 18

3 Quality of Care in the Elderly 21
3.1 Quality Assurance 21
3.2 Patient Benefit and -Risks 22

3.3 Efficacy of (New) Drugs in the Elderly 23
3.3.1 International Harmonisation on Registration of New Drugs . 23
3.3.2 Requirements for Documentation and Use in the Elderly ... 24
3.4 Evidence Based Medicine 24
3.4.1 What EBM Is 24
3.4.2 Practising EBM 25
3.4.3 Grading Evidences and Clinical Recommendations 25
3.5 Shortcomings for EBM in the Elderly 29
3.5.1 General Aspects 29
3.5.2 Documentation of Clinical Benefits 29
3.6 Organisational and Professional Aspcts 31
3.6.1 Resources, Priorities and Ethical Principles 31
3.6.2 Patient Chart Order System 33
3.6.3 Prescribing 33
3.7 Conclusions 34
References 34

4 Inappropriate Drugs in the Elderly 37
4.1 Introduction 37
4.2 Benzodiazepines 38
4.2.1 Pharmacology 39
4.2.2 Risks 39
4.2.3 Insomnia 40
4.2.4 Use and Discontinuation 41
4.3 Antipsychotic Drugs 41
4.4 NSAID 42
4.5 Drugs with Anticholinergic Effects 43
4.6 Conclusions 44
References 44

5 Drugs and Common Health Conditions in Old Age 49
5.1 Gastrointestinal Health Problems 49
5.2 Constipation 50
5.2.1 Treatment 51
5.3 Dryness of the Mouth 51
5.3.1 Risk Factors for Dryness of the Mouth 52
5.3.2 Treatment 52
5.4 Peptic Ulcers and Chronic Gastritis 53
5.4.1 Treatment 56
5.5 Hiatus Hernia 56
5.5.1 Treatment 57
5.6 Urinary Incontinence 58
5.6.1 Stress Urinary Incontinence 59
5.6.2 Overactive Bladder/Urge Incontinence 59
5.6.3 Drugs and Urinary Incontinence 61

5.7 Renal Failure in Old Age 62
5.7.1 Drugs that Can Increase the Risk of Renal Failure 62
5.8 Obstruction of Urinary Flow 64
5.9 Falls and Fractures 64
5.9.1 Fall Prevention 66
5.10 Osteoporosis 67
5.10.1 Symptoms and Signs of Osteoporosis 69
5.10.2 Treatment 69
5.11 Sarcopenia, Muscle Weakness in Old Age 70
5.12 Orthostatic Hypotension 70
5.12.1 Treatment 72
5.13 Vertigo 73
5.13.1 Treatment 74
5.14 Conclusions 75
References 76

6 Drugs and Neuro-Psychiatric Disorders 79
6.1 Introduction 79
6.2 Delirium in the Elderly 79
6.2.1 Risk Factors 81
6.2.2 Features of Delirium 82
6.2.3 Diagnosis 83
6.2.4 Treatment 83
6.3 Dementia 84
6.4 Affective Disorders 85
6.4.1 Depression 85
6.4.2 Anxiety 86
6.5 Psychotic Disease 86
6.6 Conclusions 87
References 87

7 Errors, Problems, Events and Reactions on Medication 91
7.1 Introduction 91
7.2 Medication Errors 92
7.2.1 To Err is Human 93
7.2.2 5 Million Live Campaign 94
7.3 Drug-Related Problems 95
7.4 Adverse Drug Events 95
7.5 Adverse Drug Reactions 95
7.5.1 WHO Programme for International Drug Monitoring 96
7.5.2 Pharmacovigilance and Reporting 96
7.6 Risk Medications 97
7.7 Risk Patients—The Elderly 98
7.8 Conclusions 99
References 99

8 Practical Problems Related to the Patients Medication Intake 101
8.1 Confusing Names 101
8.1.1 Original and Generic Drugs 102
8.1.2 Parallel Imported Drugs 103
8.1.3 Analogue Drugs 103
8.1.4 Other Product Names 104
8.2 Problem to Remember 104
8.3 Problem in Handling 105
8.4 Problem to Swallow 105
8.5 Food Interactions 107
8.6 Short Use Before Date 109
8.7 Conclusions 110
References 110

9 Compliance and Concordance 111
9.1 Introduction 111
9.2 From Compliance to Concordance 112
9.3 Compliance/Adherence in the Elderly 112
9.4 Clinical Consequences 113
9.5 Practical Problems 114
9.6 Knowledge, Attitudes and Motivation 114
9.7 Tools to Detect Problems Related to Non-compliance 114
9.8 Interventions for Improvement 115
9.8.1 Systematic Reviews of Strategies to Improve Compliance in the Elderly 115
9.8.2 Communicating Evidences for Benefit and Harm 116
9.8.3 Motivational Interviewing 116
9.9 Conclusions 116
References 117

10 Strategies and Interventions for Improvement 119
10.1 Introduction 119
10.2 Information Technology Development Within Health Care 120
10.3 Evidence Based Database Sources for Effective Clinical Practices 120
10.3.1 Cochrane 120
10.3.2 NICE 121
10.4 Pharmaceutical Care and Medicines Management 121
10.5 Medication Reconciliation 122
10.6 Medication Review 124
10.7 Trigger Tools 124
10.8 Personalised Medicine 125
10.9 Conclusions 125
References 126

11 Summary and Perspectives 129
11.1 Vision and Objectives for Medication Use in the Elderly 129
11.2 Quality Improvement 130
11.3 Product- or Patient- Centred Treatment 130
11.4 Summary of Simple Practice Conclusions 131
References 132

Index 133

Chapter 1
Aging and Drugs

Abstract The number of elderly is increasing in the developed part of the world. With increasing age the prevalence of many diseases will increase. This promotes high use of drugs. Pharmacotherapy can effectively cure, prevent or alleviate many conditions and improve quality of life but with aging there is an increased risk of drug-related problems. Older people are often excluded in trials, hence we often have limited knowledge regarding efficacy of pharmacotherapy in the elderly. Polypharmacy is common among elderly, which complicates pharmacotherapy since the risks of drug-drug interactions and adverse drug effects are increased.

Many different professionals and sometimes different health care providers are involved in the care of elderly. Cooperation, documentation and communication have to be improved within the professions, between professions and with the patient.

Keywords Drug-related problems · Epidemiology · Polypharmacy

1.1 Introduction

Aging is an inevitable process characterised by continuous decline in function and increased susceptibility to disease. With aging there is also a decreased ability to adapt to external changes. There are many theories explaining how the process of aging occurs. These theories include oxidative stress and various genetic mechanisms.

In this book as in most of the scientific literature, elderly is defined as 65 years or older. Chronologic age is most often used to define elderly although there are great inter-individual variations within this population. Older persons differ from younger adults in the frequency of co-morbidities and frailty. The fact that elderly often suffer from many concomitant diseases makes it harder to make correct diagnoses. Aging may also change the clinical presentation of a disease. Symptoms are more likely to be non-specific than in younger adults.

P. Midlöv et al., *Drug-Related Problems in the Elderly*,
DOI 10.1007/978-90-481-2446-6_1, © Springer Science+Business Media B.V. 2009

Due to physiological changes the ability to recover from an illness is often deteriorated, symptoms may partly remain for long time.

Elderly are more susceptible to adverse effects of drugs due to decreased physiologic reserves, polypharmacy and co-morbidity. Precribers should therefore always consider whether non-pharmacological treatment may be appropriate before prescribing additional drugs to elderly patients.

1.2 Epidemiology

The elderly represent 14% of the total population in the more developed region of the world and this proportion is expected to increase to 23% in 2030 (United Nations 1999).

In Europe the number of elderly has increased during the last forty years and this demographic development is predicted to continue in the coming years (Council of Europe 2003). Rates of mortality improvement have accelerated over the last 100 years. Much of the rise in life expectancy is due to reductions in death rates at younger ages, but death rates are now also declining among the elderly. Approximately half of female and a third of male deaths occur after age 80 in developed countries (Kannisto et al. 1994).

These changes in demography will of course have impact on health care since age is a risk factor for many diseases. Dementia, cardio-vascular disease, diabetes, and cancer are some examples of diseases with increasing prevalence with age, hence the number of patients with these conditions will also increase. This promotes high use of medications in older people. Frail elderly people often use many drugs, in particular those elderly residing in nursing homes. These patients are most susceptible to adverse effects from drugs.

1.3 Drug-Related Problems

Pharmacotherapy can effectively improve quality of life, cure, and prevent or alleviate symptoms in many conditions in late life. Drugs are however powerful and must be handled appropriately. This is especially important for elderly patients. Adverse effects and other drug-related problems (DRPs) are common in elderly patients (Hanlon et al. 2003). Drug-related problem has been defined as "an event or circumstance involving drug treatment that actually or potentially interferes with a patient's experiencing an optimum outcome of medical care" (Hepler and Strand 1990). With this definition DRP include e.g. drug use without an indication, drug interactions, subtherapeutic dosage, overdosage, noncompliance, drug interactions and adverse drug reactions (ADRs). Therapeutic failure may be due to underuse of medications. Reasons for this could be lack of patient adherence but also suboptimal prescribing. All medications have risk of adverse effects with varying clinical consequences and severity. These adverse effects can result from medications taken individually or can result from pharmacokinetic and pharmacodynamic interactions of medications used in combination. Elderly patients are more susceptible to ADR than younger patients. This is due to the fact that elderly use many drugs but also due to physiological changes with increasing age that affects the pharmacokinetics and pharmacodynamics. However, in the absence of disease, the decline in physiological functions most often causes no symptoms. The potential risk of drug-drug interactions is increased with the number of drugs used and age. Since the interactions are more common in frail patients, the consequences are likely to be worse than in younger individuals. If the prescriber is aware of potential interactions these can many times be avoided by choosing other drugs. If this is not possible, drug dosages have to be adjusted and pharmacotherapy more cautiously evaluated. Adverse drug reactions are common preventable causes of emergency medical admissions in the elderly (Chan et al. 2001). It is not only ADRs that might cause problems in the elderly but also withdrawal events. Adverse drug withdrawal events are related to the removal of a drug.

Hospitalisation accounts for a great part of total cost of care. Studies have shown that 15–22% of the hospitalised elderly patients are admitted because of DRP (Bero et al. 1991, Roughead et al. 1998, Cooper 1999). Also it is reported that the majority of adverse drug reactions in the elderly can be prevented (Beijer and de Blaey 2002). It has further been shown that the majority of hospitalised patients have DRPs (Blix et al. 2004). Use of unnecessary drugs is quite frequent among elderly and one quarter of these unnecessary drugs are started during hospitalisation (Hajjar et al. 2005). Drug-related problems may increase the need for hospital care and also have impact on mortality. Adverse drug effects are between the fourth and sixth leading causes of death in USA (Lazarou et al. 1998).

There is also a financial aspect on drug-related problems. For every dollar spent on drugs in US nursing homes facilities, 1.33 dollars in health care resources are consumed in the treatment of drug-related problems (Bootman et al. 1997).

Drug-related problems thus cause much suffering for the elderly patients and great costs for the society. The good thing on the other hand is that these drug-related problems often are preventable. In this book we describe the physiological changes that make elderly more susceptible to adverse effects. There is special focus on medications that are considered to be inappropriate for elderly patients. These medications include long-acting benzodiazepines and antipsychotic drugs. Different conditions that are common among elderly are covered. We will also describe problems due to organisational shortcomings.

1.4 Evidence Based Medicine

Many new drugs have been developed for diseases with increasing prevalence. The main users of these drugs, i.e. the elderly patients, are not always included in trials of these drugs (Bugeja et al. 1997, Bayer and Tadd 2000). We therefore often have limited knowledge regarding efficacy of pharmacotherapy in the elderly. In other words there is often inadequate scientific evidence about pharmacotherapy in old age. The subjects and patients in trials are often not the patients who will get the drugs in clinical practice. In reality these patients are older, have more and different diseases, more medications with the potential to affect the outcome of the treatment, more adverse effects and also a lower compliance to the treatment. In clinical trials the patients have better support including closer, more systematic and more supportive contacts with health care. The patients, in trials, feel more selected and prioritised. For professionals in health care it is difficult to generalise results from trials to elderly patients.

1.5 Polypharmacy

There is no universal definition of polypharmacy. One common definition is the use of five or more drugs. This is also the definition that we use in this book. With increasing number of drugs the risk for adverse drug reactions increases.

Polypharmacy is widespread in the population, especially among the elderly (Bjerrum et al. 1998). The concomitant use of several drugs increases the risks of ADR, interactions and incorrect drug use (LeSage 1991), thus increases the risk of DRP and drug-related costs. There is also a clear relation between falling and the use of higher number of medications (Tinetti 2003). Reducing polypharmacy is not always easy. Elderly often have diseases that require pharmacotherapy. In a Finnish study they achieved some drug reductions but when the intervention ceased the number of drugs used soon returned to its earlier level (Pitkala et al. 2001).

With more knowledge of drug-related problems in the elderly, systematic medication review has become more common. The objective is not primarily to reduce the number of drugs but to achieve a more optimal pharmacotherapy and reduce the number of drug-related problems. Clinicians who try to reduce polypharmacy need to exercise caution in stopping medications in the elderly. In that case medications can often be successfully stopped without causing an adverse drug withdrawal event (ADWE) (Graves et al. 1997). It is recommended to stop one medication at a time. In an American study the number of medications discontinued was significantly associated with ADWE occurrence (Graves et al. 1997).

It is also important to improve patients' knowledge about their medicines since medication beliefs is a strong predictor of adherence (Horne and Weinman 1999). Thus if the patient knows what medication is used, the reason for pharmacotherapy, and believe in the benefit then adherence will be improved.

1.6 General Improved Quality

For improved quality in the use of medications in the society and for the individual patients we need to identify problems and errors in structures and in processes to improve the outcome of care and to reduce errors (Donobedian 2003). In most industrial countries we have reasonable good structures for care. We have suitable diagnostic tools, medications and trained physicians, nurses, pharmacists and paramedics. We need to improve the process of care. Documentation and communication of prescribed drugs is very important within the health care system and also for use and follow-up on the effects of prescribing in individual patients. Cooperation, documentation and communication have to be improved within the professions, between professions and with the patient.

The main process (Fig. 1.1) for the care of a patient is normally the Primary care process (the patient handles their own drugs)—or the community care process (the patient gets help from community nurses at home or at a nursing home). All other processes such as hospital care (secondary/tertiary care) and the pharmacy process must support the main patient process. For improvement we must focus on patient safety and reduce drug-related problems. This means correct prescription and correct use (follow-up, documentation and communication) from the supportive process to the main process.

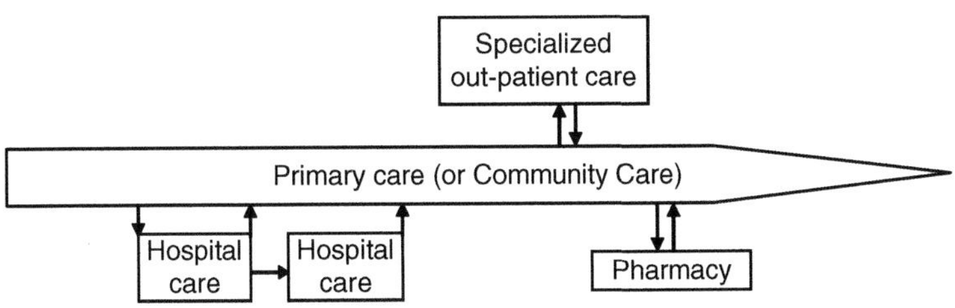

Fig. 1.1 Time scale of the patient medication processes. Main (primary care) and some important supportive processes

Especially for the elderly this means for example improved:

- Documentation of medicinal product on benefits and harm in elderly with complicating other diseases and circumstances
- Electronic support system for correct prescription, documentation and communication.
- Documentation of aims and treatment results for each patient
- Documentation and communication of relevant patient care aspects and medications within health care
- Communication with patients/careers on therapeutic options, decisions and potential problems

1.7 Specific Problems, Consequences, and Improvements

This book focuses on specific problems with medication and provides a background and consequences of drug use, with focus on the elderly. For most problems we also provide suggestions for help, and improvement (Table 1.1).

Table 1.1 Some drug-related problems and potential solutions presented in this book

Problem	Potential solutions
Drug-related problems and medication errors	Risk Medication, Medication Review, Medication Reconciliation, Adverse Drug Events, Trigger tools.
Wrong drug or dose	Training of prescribers but also all staff in the elderly care, Evidence Based Medicine, Computerised Prescriber Order Entry, Educational Outreach, inappropriate medications, documentation of clinical benefits, risk medications, drug interactions, pharmacological alterations with age.
Compliance	Identification of the patient's problems, empowerment, cooperation, documentation and communication within the professions, between professions and with the patient.

1.8 Conclusions

- The number of elderly is increasing in the developed world
- Knowledge about efficacy of drugs in the elderly is limited
- Drug-related problems are common in the elderly
- These drug-related problems have impact on morbidity, mortality and costs

References

Bayer A and Tadd W (2000) Unjustified exclusion of elderly people from studies submitted to research ethics committee for approval: descriptive study. BMJ 321(7267): 992–993

Beijer HJ and de Blaey CJ (2002) Hospitalisations caused by adverse drug reactions (ADR): a meta-analysis of observational studies. Pharm World Sci 24(2): 46–54

Bero LA, Lipton HL, Bird JA (1991) Characterization of geriatric drug-related hospital readmissions. Med Care 29(10): 989–1003

Bjerrum L, Sogaard J, Hallas J et al. (1998) Polypharmacy: correlations with sex, age and drug regimen. A prescription database study. Eur J Clin Pharmacol 54(3): 197–202

Blix HS, Viktil KK, Reikvam A et al. (2004) The majority of hospitalised patients have drug-related problems: results from a prospective study in general hospitals. Eur J Clin Pharmacol 60(9): 651–658

Bootman JL, Harrison DL, Cox E (1997) The health care cost of drug-related morbidity and mortality in nursing facilities. Arch Intern Med 157(18): 2089–2096

Bugeja G, Kumar A, Banerjee AK (1997) Exclusion of elderly people from clinical research: a descriptive study of published reports. BMJ 315(7115): 1059

Chan M, Nicklason F, Vial JH (2001) Adverse drug events as a cause of hospital admission in the elderly. Intern Med J 31(4): 199–205

Cooper JW (1999) Adverse drug reaction-related hospitalizations of nursing facility patients: a 4-year study. South Med J 92(5): 485–490

Council of Europe (2003) Recent demographic developments in Europe. Strasbourg, Council of Europe Publishing

Donobedian A (2003) An introduction to quality assurance in health care. Oxford University Press, New York

Graves T, Hanlon JT, Schmader KE et al. (1997) Adverse events after discontinuing medications in elderly outpatients. Arch Intern Med 157(19): 2205–2210

Hajjar ER, Hanlon JT, Sloane RJ et al. (2005) Unnecessary drug use in frail older people at hospital discharge. J Am Geriatr Soc 53(9): 1518–1523

Hanlon JT, Lindblad CI, Hajjar ER et al. (2003) Update on drug-related problems in the elderly. Am J Geriatr Pharmacother 1(1): 38–43

Hepler CD and Strand LM (1990) Opportunities and responsibilities in pharmaceutical care. Am J Hosp Pharm 47(3): 533–543

Horne R and Weinman J (1999) Patients' beliefs about prescribed medicines and their role in adherence to treatment in chronic physical illness. J Psychosom Res 47(6): 555–567

Kannisto V, Lauritsen J, Thatcher AR et al. (1994) Reductions in mortality at advanced age: several decades of evidence from 27 countries. Population and development review 20(4): 793–810

Lazarou J, Pomeranz BH, Corey PN (1998) Incidence of adverse drug reactions in hospitalized patients: a meta- analysis of prospective studies. JAMA 279(15): 1200–1205

LeSage J (1991) Polypharmacy in geriatric patients. Nurs Clin North Am 26(2): 273–290

Pitkala KH, Strandberg TE, Tilvis RS (2001) Is it possible to reduce polypharmacy in the elderly? A randomised, controlled trial. Drugs Aging 18(2): 143–149

Roughead EE, Gilbert AL, Primrose JG et al. (1998) Drug-related hospital admissions: a review of Australian studies published 1988–1996. Med J Aust 168(8): 405–408

Tinetti ME (2003) Clinical practice. Preventing falls in elderly persons. N Engl J Med 348(1): 42–49

United Nations (1999) World population prospects: The 1998 revision. United Nations Secretariat, Department of Economic and Social Affairs, Population Division, New York

Chapter 2
Physiological Alterations with Aging

Abstract Elderly are more susceptible to adverse drug reactions than younger persons. This is partly due to age-related physiological changes that affect pharmacodynamics and pharmacokinetics. An understanding of these age-related changes and of the pharmacokinetics of individual drugs is important before prescribing drugs to elderly patients. The most frequent and important change affecting pharmacokinetics is the decline in renal elimination. A disability to excrete drugs is an important consequence of the impaired kidney function that occurs in old age and it increases the risk of drug-accumulation and adverse drug reactions. Pharmacodynamical changes affect most organs since the older patients have impaired homeostatic mechanisms.

Other important factors for the increased risk of adverse drug reactions are polypharmacy and multimorbidity. Before adding a drug the physician should try to diagnose the condition and rule out drugs as the cause of the problem. When a drug is added the dose should be lower than in younger adults and then the dose can be titrated to a therapeutic response.

Keywords Pharmacokinetics · Pharmacodynamics · Drug-drug interactions · Adverse drug reactions

2.1 Introduction

The clinical response to medication depends on pharmacokinetic and pharmacodynamic conditions. Elderly are because of pharmacological alterations more susceptible to drug-related problem (DRP) (Turnheim 2004). A clear relationship is evident between old age and the risk of adverse drug reaction (Bordet et al. 2001). There are different explanations for older adults' vulnerability. The body of young adults has great physiologic reserve in the function of most organs. Already in early adulthood physiological changes that may affect medications begin. For older adults the reserve is diminished, i.e. aging results in a reduction in homeostatic mechanisms. This leads to increased vulnerability to disease and susceptibility to drugs. Decline of physiological functions is a gradual ongoing process. An abrupt decline in any function is always due to disease or external causes, such as drugs, and not to

P. Midlöv et al., *Drug-Related Problems in the Elderly*,
DOI 10.1007/978-90-481-2446-6_2,

normal aging. The inter-individual variability is greater in elderly than in younger adults. Individuals become more dissimilar as they age. Individual physiologic characteristics are probably more important than chronologic age in predicting effects of pharmacotherapy. Age, disease, current and previous drug use as well as genetics are some factors that may influence the function and susceptibility to drugs.

Some healthy elderly may not be very affected by pharmacological alterations whereas others have become very susceptible to adverse effects of drugs. It is especially important for elderly patients that pharmacotherapy is individualised. With knowledge of expected physiologic changes with aging, decisions should be based on the individual patient's disease and concomitant medications.

2.2 Pharmacokinetics

The bioavailability of a drug, taken orally, depends on many factors, including absorption through the gastrointestinal mucosa and liver function. For most drugs information on pharmacokinetics refers mostly to patients younger than 65 years, despite the fact that it is mainly elderly persons who will use these drugs (Perucca 2007). It is important to be aware of age-depending differences in pharmacokinetics between younger and older adults. To prevent accumulation of a drug when its clearance is reduced the prescriber can reduce the dose or increase dosage interval. All steps in pharmacokinetics may be affected in the elderly (Table 2.1).

2.2.1 Absorption of Drugs

Drugs can be administered in different ways. The most common and important way is orally. Most medications are passively absorbed and aging does not affect this absorption to any significant extent. The absorption of orally taken drugs depends on the function of ventricle, intestines, and the blood flow to the intestines. Although old age is characterised by slowing of gastric emptying, and decreased peristalsis, in the absence of malabsorptive disease, absorption of most drugs is not diminished with age (Turnheim 2003). Diseases affecting the gastrointestinal organs can of course affect absorption. Food intake may also affect absorption of drugs as described in Chapter 8.

The absorption rate of drugs administered as intramuscular or subcutaneous injections may be affected in elderly because of reduced tissue blood perfusion. This is also true for transdermal administration, e.g. patches and gels, of drugs (Turnheim 2003).

2.2.2 Distribution of Drugs

When a drug has been absorbed it enters the systemic circulation and gets distributed throughout the body. The volume of distribution is the theoretical space in a patient that a substance occupies. This is influenced by the proportions of lean body mass versus fat. There is a decline in fat-free mass and body water, whereas there is an

Table 2.1 Physiological alterations with aging that may affect pharmacotherapy

Pharmacokinetic	Change	Change due to	Clinical importance	Drugs that may be affected (examples)
Absorption	May be slowed but the amount absorbed is mostly not affected	Decreased function of ventricle, intestines and the blood flow to thc intestines	Little	
Distribution	Decrease in the volume of distribution of hydrophilic drugs and increase in the volume of distribution of lipophilic drugs	Decline in fat-free mass and increase in body fat with aging	Important for some drugs	Diazepam and flunitrazepam may have increased plasma half-life. Water soluble drugs as digoxin and teophylline have higher peak plasma concentrations and shorter half-lives
Metabolism	Hepatic metabolism may be reduced	Decreased hepatic blood flow. Decreased liver mass. Diminished enzymatic function	Important for some drugs	Verapamil and teophylline
Renal elimination	Renal elimination is reduced	Decline in glomerular filtration Decreased renal blood flow	Very important for many drugs	Lithium, digoxin, ranitidine, metformin

increase in body fat with age (Vestal 1997, Kyle et al. 2001, Turnheim 2004). The increase in body fat is relatively greater for men than women. Women however have a lower lean body mass than men at all ages. The increase in percentage of body fat and the reduction in total body water result in changes in the distribution of drugs depending on lipid solubility. The half-life of a drug increases with the volume of distribution. With a decrease in the volume of distribution of hydrophilic drugs, these drugs have higher peak plasma concentrations and shorter half-life in the elderly. This is true for drugs as digoxin and teophylline and may result in toxic plasma concentrations for doses that would not be toxic to younger adults.

Since the volume of distribution is increased, the elimination half-life of lipid-soluble drugs is increased. This affects for example medium- and long-acting benzodiazepines as well as i.e. verapamil that can accumulate in the body.

The elimination half-life ($t_{1/2}$) is determined by the volume of distribution (V_d), divided by its clearance (Cl); $t_{1/2} = 0.693 \times V_d / Cl$

The elimination half life of a drug will thus increase if the volume of distribution is increased as for lipophilic drugs in the elderly or if the clearance is affected, the latter mainly hepatic metabolism or renal excretion.

Muscle mass decrease with age (Kyle et al. 2001). For drugs that are bound to muscle tissue, i.e. digoxin, this may result in higher plasma-concentrations.

Some drugs are bound to plasma proteins in blood. Plasma protein levels in blood may be decreased in the elderly, but this is most often not clinically relevant since a drug's elimination increases when the free, unbound drug concentration is enhanced (Turnheim 1998). The plasma albumin level may however be markedly decreased in elderly suffering from malnutrition or severe disease. For those patients the concentration of the free unbound drug can reach toxic levels (Walter-Sack and Klotz 1996).

Very old individuals often loose weight. There is thus a risk that these patients receive higher doses per unit bodyweight than younger heavier patients (Turnheim 2003).

2.2.3 Metabolism

The liver is the most important site of metabolism for many medications. Metabolism of drugs depends on hepatic blood flow and with aging hepatic blood flow and liver mass is decreased. Metabolism also depends on the function and capacity of drug-metabolising enzymes in the liver. The most important enzymes are those within the cytochrome p450-system. These enzymes, i.e. CYP3A4 and CYP2D6 may be of different capacity due to genetic differences. Both the enzymatic function and the hepatic blood flow may be diminished with increased age but the hepatic metabolism of drugs is mostly not much affected even if there are great inter-individual differences (Turnheim 2003). It may be difficult to predict changes in hepatic metabolism for the individual patient. The clearance of flow-limited drugs is correlated with the age-related reduction in blood flow whereas there is no age-related reduction in clearance of capacity-limited drugs (Le Couteur and McLean 1998). Flow-limited drugs with reported reductions in systematic clearance in elderly are e.g. propranolol, chlomethiazole, and morphine (Woodhouse and James 1990). There are many things besides age that have impact on metabolism of drugs. Concomitant medications and diseases are factors that further affect drug metabolism in the liver. The nutritional status of a patient has effect on the rate of drug metabolism. In frail elderly, drug metabolism is diminished to a greater extent than in elderly with normal body weight (Walter-Sack and Klotz 1996, Vestal 1997).

2.2.4 Renal Elimination

Elderly people's capacity to concentrate the urine decreases, which results in that they need larger amounts of urine to secrete the same amount of toxic waste products compared with younger adults.

Most drugs, including metabolites, are eliminated via the kidneys. Before renal elimination many drugs are metabolised to more water-soluble metabolites. There is a continuous decline in renal function with aging. Kidney mass is substantially reduced in old age (Beck 1998). The decline in renal function is both due to decreased Glomerular Filtration Rate (GFR) and decreased renal blood flow. The absolute most important change with age is the decline in glomerular filtration. The Glomerular filtration rate declines by approximately 25–50% between the ages of 20 and 90 (Turnheim 2003). This is a progressive decline that continues throughout life. Aging is also associated with the development of glomerulosclerosis and interstitial fibrosis (Muhlberg and Platt 1999).

Serum creatinine is not a good measure of renal function in elderly because muscle mass is reduced and the production of creatinine is thus reduced. Estimation of GFR based on serum creatinine is therefore not accurate enough in the elderly (Baracskay et al. 1997). Creatinine clearance should be used instead. Another possibility is measurement of cystatin C in plasma. The rate of production of cystatin C is relatively constant so it seems to be a more reliable estimation of GFR also in older adults.

Due to the decrease in renal function the prescriber should always adjust drug dosages according to renal function. The decline in renal function increase the risk for adverse drug reactions (Muhlberg and Platt 1999). Renal function is however often overlooked when prescribing renally excreted drugs to older patients (Papaioannou et al. 2000). Many drugs are excreted fully or to a greater part by the kidneys. For drugs with narrow therapeutic indices and that are renally eliminated e.g. digoxin, metformin and lithium, it is especially important to adjust and monitor treatment. Renal function is however important for the elimination of many other drugs as well. One should also remember that many diseases with increasing prevalence in old age influence renal function in addition to age-related changes. Diabetes and hypertension are two common diseases that may further decrease renal function. A disability to excrete drugs is an important consequence of the impaired kidney function that occurs in old age and it increases the risk of drug-accumulation and adverse drug reactions. Especially with additional diseases the consequences for the renal function and the risk of drug-related problems increase.

2.2.5 Water and Electrolyte Balance

The activity of the renin-angiotensin system is reduced with age (Muhlberg and Platt 1999). The ability of the kidney to concentrate urine maximally after water deprivation decreases with age, as does the ability to excrete a water and salt load, particularly during the night. Nocturnal polyuria is common in the elderly (Lubran 1995). Diuretics are commonly used in the elderly. There is an increased risk for hypokalemia and hyponatremia from diuretics in the elderly (Passare et al. 2004). Electrolyte disturbances may also be caused by several types of drugs in the elderly and it is important to monitor serum electrolyte levels in the elderly. Treatment with diuretics may cause discomfort due to polyuria. This and the risk of electrolyte disturbances and other ADRs are reasons for continuous reassessment of treatment with diuretics.

Acute renal failure due to NSAIDs is usually due to prerenal causes but may be caused by acute interstitial nephritis. Usually the worsening in renal function does not depend on dose (Muhlberg and Platt 1999). Use of NSAID is thus risky and may affect the elimination of concomitant medications.

2.3 Pharmacodynamics

The pharmacodynamic effect of a drug depends on the concentration of the drug at the receptor, the response at the receptor and homeostatic mechanisms. Age-related changes in pharmacodynamics may occur at the receptor or signal-transduction level. A third possibility is that homeostatic mechanisms may be attenuated (Turnheim 2003). Pharmacodynamic changes with aging are more difficult to study than pharmacokinetic changes and there is little evidence of the mechanism underlying pharmacodynamic changes. Many measures of response are subjective and may be influenced by several factors. Comparison of pharmacodynamic in young adults and elderly may be hard due to baseline differences.

Most organ systems are more vulnerable in the elderly. In general this means an increased sensitivity to unwanted effects of drugs.

2.3.1 Cardiovascular Effects

One of the few examples of decreased susceptibility among elderly is the effect of catecholamines on the heart. There is a down-regulation of beta-adrenergic receptors and a reduced response to beta-adrenergic stimulation (Turnheim 1998). This results in decreased effect of betablockers on heart rate and stroke volume. In the elderly betablockers may be less effective than other drugs against hypertension and they should not be considered appropriate for first-line therapy of uncomplicated hypertension in the elderly (Grossman and Messerli 2002).

Many other changes make older adults more vulnerable regarding cardiovascular drugs. There is a decrease in baroreceptor reflex response. This may explain the increased sensitivity to nitrates (Marchionni et al. 1990). With age there is a loss of blood vessel distensibility and enhanced intimal thickness. This can partly explain the increase of systolic blood pressure. Aging is also associated with a reduction in baroreflex-mediated heart rate response to hypotensive stimuli (Verhaeverbeke and Mets 1997, Lakatta and Levy 2003).

Postural hypotension contributes to the risk of syncope and falls especially in the elderly (Verhaeverbeke and Mets 1997). In case of postural hypotension, drug treatment should always be reviewed. Due to a decrease in homeostatic mechanisms elderly more often have postural hypotension from drugs that lower blood pressure than younger patients (Turnheim 1998). It is not only cardiovascular drugs that may cause postural hypotension, i.e. many antipsychotic drugs and drugs for Parkinson's disease may also cause this adverse effect. Elevated blood pressure play however an important role in the development of brain complications of hypertension and reduction of abnormally elevated blood pressure safely and effectively decreases morbidity and mortality rates in the elderly (Amenta et al. 2002).

Increased age is most likely associated with enhanced susceptibility to digoxin toxicity, possibly due to unknown pharmacodynamic changes, even when plasma concentrations are within therapeutic range (Miura et al. 2000).

Elderly patients often exhibit an enhanced dose response to warfarin (Hylek 2001). With the knowledge of high risk for serious adverse drug reactions from warfarin, thorough monitoring of treatment is mandatory.

2.3.2 Central Nervous System

The pharmacodynamics are affected due to altered levels of neurotransmitters and receptors in the central nervous system with age. The blood-brain barrier may be less effective, hence the brain may be exposed to higher drug and toxin levels in elderly subjects (Toornvliet et al. 2006).

There is an increased risk of sedation and delirium with increased age. There is also an increased risk of antidopaminergic effects such as parkinsonism due to antipsychotic drugs. Many other drugs that pass the blood-brain barrier may cause adverse effects in the elderly. The response of opioids may be increased in the elderly, resulting in oversedation (Turnheim 1998).

Treatment of epilepsy is often more complex in the elderly (Tallis et al. 2002). Plasma concentration of antiepileptic drugs that are adequate for younger patients may be toxic for older adults. Clinical response, and not only plasma concentration of the drug, is more important in the elderly for evaluation of antiepileptic treatment.

2.4 Drug-Drug Interactions

The probability of a drug-drug interaction increases with the number of drugs used and age (Seymour and Routledge 1998, Veehof et al. 2000, Doubova Dubova et al. 2007). Drug-drug interactions are a risk factor for ADR (Mackinnon and Helper 2003). This is especially important for drugs with narrow therapeutic margin such as digoxin, warfarin, carbamazepine, and lithium. Most often drug-drug interactions are predictable and thus an important cause of preventable adverse drug reactions. Many hospital admissions of elderly patients occur after administration of drugs known to cause drug-drug interactions and are thus preventable (Juurlink et al. 2003). Elderly use more medications and are therefore at greater risk of drug-drug interaction. It is well proven that drug-drug interactions have negative effects on morbidity. It is important to be aware of possible drug-drug interactions and try to avoid them or at least adjust drug dosages. In Table 2.2 some common drug-drug interactions in the elderly are presented.

Table 2.2 Examples of common drug-drug interactions

Drug 1	Drug 2	Potential outcome
ACE-inhibitors	Spironolactone	Hyperkalemia
ACE-inhibitors	NSAID	Hyperkalemia, decline in renal function
Aspirin	NSAID	Increased risk for peptic ulcer
Ciprofloxacin	Olanzapine	Ciprofloxacin inhibits CYP1A2. As a result the plasma-concentration of olanzapine increases
Dextropropoxyphene	Carbamazepine	Increased plasma-concentration of carbamazepine
Digoxin	Furosemide	Hypokalemia may increase risk for digitalis-intoxication
Verapamil	Atenolol	Bradycardia and hypotension

2.5 Drug-Disease Interactions

The great inter-individual variability in susceptibility to drugs among elderly is at least partly explained by differences in multi-morbidity. Diseases that affect renal function make the patient more susceptible to ADR due to reduction in renal elimination. Diseases affecting the Central Nervous System make that individual at higher risk of ADR from the CNS than healthier adults of the same age. In the same way diseases that affect other organ systems may make elderly even more susceptible to drugs. In Table 2.3 some common drug-disease interactions in the elderly are presented.

Table 2.3 Examples of common drug-disease interactions

Drug	Disease	Potential outcome
Anticholinergic drugs	Dementia	Delirium
Antipsychotics	Parkinson's disease (PD)	Worsening of PD symptoms
NSAID	Decreased renal function	Renal failure
NSAID	Heart failure	Worsening of heart failure
Thiazides	Gout	Worsening of gout
Tricyclic antidepressants (TCAs)	Epilepsy	Lower seizure threshold (more so if toxic levels of TCA)

2.6 Adverse Drug Reactions

All drugs may cause adverse drug reactions (ADRs). These adverse effects are either unpredictable (hyper-sensitivity) or dose-depending. The risk of ADR is increased for several reasons in the elderly. The physiological alterations, the high number of medications and concomitant diseases increase the risk of ADR. This is further described in Chapter 7. The symptoms may be harder to detect since they may be misinterpreted as symptoms from a disease. The diagnosis of ADR may be difficult and sometimes mislabelled as normal aging. Drug-induced fatigue or delirium may be undiagnosed as ADR and instead just attributed to old age.

The number of medications increases the risk of ADR (Gurwitz et al. 2005). Medication errors at all levels also increase risk of ADR. These errors are e.g. wrong dosage or wrong medication (commission error). It has further been shown that transfer of elderly patients between different care levels increases the risk of ADR (Cooper 1999).

It is important to be aware of the possibility that adverse effects can occur with drugs and drug doses unlikely to produce adverse effects in young adults. Symptoms that should be evaluated as possible adverse drug reactions in older patients include delirium, syncope and dehydration. Adverse drug reactions occur frequently in elderly and are often preventable. In a study on patients in two long-term care facilities it was found that serious, more life-threatening, and fatal adverse drug reactions were more likely to be preventable than were less severe events (Gurwitz et al. 2005). Many severe ADRs can thus be avoided with closer monitoring and thorough evaluation of drug use.

Adverse drug reactions are mostly dose related and therefore it is important to choose the lowest dose required for beneficial effect.

2.7 Adverse Drug Withdrawal Events

It is important to be aware of possible adverse drug withdrawal events (ADWE). These events may be caused by physiological withdrawal reaction, but it is also possible that the underlying disease is worsened. An example of ADWE is delirium or seizures that may occur after abrupt discontinuing of benzodiazepines or alcohol.

There are not many studies on ADWE. In one study the authors found that ADWEs were common in nursing home residents (Gerety et al. 1993). Multiple medications and multiple diagnoses increased the risk for ADWE. To avoid ADWE it is advisable to withdraw one drug at a time and evaluate the outcome. If possible it is best to go slow both when initiating and discontinuing pharmacotherapy in the elderly. Knowledge about ADWE is often sparse and this could be helped by drug discontinuation guidelines.

2.8 Conclusions

- There are many physiological changes with aging that make elderly more susceptible to drugs
- The most important change affecting pharmacokinetics is the decline in renal function
- Elderly have impaired homeostatic mechanisms
- Due to these changes most organs are more vulnerable in the elderly
- There is an increased risk of adverse drug reactions and adverse drug withdrawal events in old age

References

Amenta F, Mignini F, Rabbia F et al. (2002) Protective effect of anti-hypertensive treatment on cognitive function in essential hypertension: analysis of published clinical data. J Neurol Sci 203–204: 147–151

Baracskay D, Jarjoura D, Cugino A et al. (1997) Geriatric renal function: estimating glomerular filtration in an ambulatory elderly population. Clin Nephrol 47(4): 222–228

Beck LH (1998) Changes in renal function with aging. Clin Geriatr Med 14(2): 199–209

Bordet R, Gautier S, Le Louet H et al. (2001) Analysis of the direct cost of adverse drug reactions in hospitalised patients. Eur J Clin Pharmacol 56(12): 935–941

Cooper JW (1999) Adverse drug reaction-related hospitalizations of nursing facility patients: a 4-year study. South Med J 92(5): 485–490

Doubova Dubova SV, Reyes-Morales H, Torres-Arreola Ldel P et al. (2007) Potential drug-drug and drug-disease interactions in prescriptions for ambulatory patients over 50 years of age in family medicine clinics in Mexico City. BMC Health Serv Res 7: 147

Gerety MB, Cornell JE, Plichta DT et al. (1993) Adverse events related to drugs and drug withdrawal in nursing home residents. J Am Geriatr Soc 41(12): 1326–1332

Grossman E and Messerli FH (2002) Why beta-blockers are not cardioprotective in elderly patients with hypertension. Curr Cardiol Rep 4(6): 468–473

Gurwitz JH, Field TS, Judge J et al. (2005) The incidence of adverse drug events in two large academic long-term care facilities. Am J Med 118(3): 251–258

Hylek EM (2001) Oral anticoagulants. Pharmacologic issues for use in the elderly. Clin Geriatr Med 17(1): 1–13

Juurlink DN, Mamdani M, Kopp A et al. (2003) Drug-drug interactions among elderly patients hospitalized for drug toxicity. JAMA 289(13): 1652–1658

Kyle UG, Genton L, Hans D et al. (2001) Age-related differences in fat-free mass, skeletal muscle, body cell mass and fat mass between 18 and 94 years. Eur J Clin Nutr 55(8): 663–672

Lakatta EG and Levy D (2003) Arterial and cardiac aging: major shareholders in cardiovascular disease enterprises: Part I: aging arteries: a "set up" for vascular disease. Circulation 107(1): 139–146

Le Couteur DG and McLean AJ (1998) The aging liver. Drug clearance and an oxygen diffusion barrier hypothesis. Clin Pharmacokinet 34(5): 359–373

Lubran MM (1995) Renal function in the elderly. Ann Clin Lab Sci 25(2): 122–133

Mackinnon NJ and Helper CD (2003) Indicators of preventable drug-related morbidity in older adults 2. Use within a managed care organization. J Manag Care Pharm 9(2): 134–141

Marchionni N, Ferrucci L, Fumagalli S et al. (1990) Age-related changes in the pharmacodynamics of intravenous glyceryl trinitrate. Aging (Milano) 2(1): 59–64

Miura T, Kojima R, Sugiura Y et al. (2000) Effect of aging on the incidence of digoxin toxicity. Ann Pharmacother 34(4): 427–432

Muhlberg W and Platt D (1999) Age-dependent changes of the kidneys: pharmacological implications. Gerontology 45(5): 243–253

Papaioannou A, Clarke JA, Campbell G et al. (2000) Assessment of adherence to renal dosing guidelines in long-term care facilities. J Am Geriatr Soc 48(11): 1470–1473

Passare G, Viitanen M, Torring O et al. (2004) Sodium and potassium disturbances in the elderly: prevalence and association with drug use. Clin Drug Investig 24(9): 535–544

Perucca E (2007) Age-related changes in pharmacokinetics: predictability and assessment methods. Int Rev Neurobiol 81: 183–199

Seymour RM and Routledge PA (1998) Important drug-drug interactions in the elderly. Drugs Aging 12(6): 485–494

Tallis R, Boon P, Perucca E et al. (2002) Epilepsy in elderly people: management issues. Epileptic Disord 4(Suppl 2): S33–S39

Toornvliet R, van Berckel BN, Luurtsema G et al. (2006) Effect of age on functional P-glycoprotein in the blood-brain barrier measured by use of (R)-[(11)C]verapamil and positron emission tomography. Clin Pharmacol Ther 79(6): 540–548

Turnheim K (1998) Drug dosage in the elderly. Is it rational? Drugs Aging 13(5): 357–379
Turnheim K (2003) When drug therapy gets old: pharmacokinetics and pharmacodynamics in the elderly. Exp Gerontol 38(8): 843–853
Turnheim K (2004) Drug therapy in the elderly. Exp Gerontol 39(11–12): 1731–1738
Walter-Sack I and Klotz U (1996) Influence of diet and nutritional status on drug metabolism. Clin Pharmacokinet 31(1): 47–64
Veehof L, Stewart R, Haaijer-Ruskamp F et al. (2000) The development of polypharmacy. A longitudinal study. Fam Pract 17(3): 261–267
Verhaeverbeke I and Mets T (1997) Drug-induced orthostatic hypotension in the elderly: avoiding its onset. Drug Saf 17(2): 105–118
Vestal RE (1997) Aging and pharmacology. Cancer 80(7): 1302–1310
Woodhouse KW and James OF (1990) Hepatic drug metabolism and ageing. Br Med Bull 46(1): 22–35

Chapter 3
Quality of Care in the Elderly

Abstract Quality of care is complicated, especially in the elderly. For a start we need drugs with evidence for the benefits and risks in the elderly, this is currently not always the case. Thereafter we need to use the drugs in an evidence based way, which may be difficult in the complex health care system. To achieve maximum benefit for the patient (outcome) and society (health-economy) a well planned process is needed. This includes; identification, prevention and resolving of the patients drug-related problems decisions and selection of treatment, communication and decisions together with the patient, risk minimisation, and communication within health care. Several of these aspects are presented in this chapter.

Keywords Quality · Benefits · Risks · Evidence based medicine

3.1 Quality Assurance

Quality assurance is defined by Donaobedian as "all actions taken to establish, protect, promote, and improve the quality of health care" (Donobedian 2003). He describes quality of care as an attribute of a system (structure), a set of organized activities (process), and an outcome that results from both. The definitions are described in Table 3.1. It should be noted that the efficacy of a drug (the ability for improvement under the most favourable circumstances) is included in the structure and that the effectiveness of a drug (real improvement in the care) is included in the process.

Quality can not be guaranteed. One can increase the probability that a care is "good" or "better". If the different components in the structure and process are improved the probability of a better patient outcome is increased. Sometimes it is not possible to measure patient outcomes. Instead surrogate outcomes of the process performance can be used especially if there is evidences for a link to real patient outcomes. For improvement and assessing improvement Donobedian suggests a mix of approaches in the structure, process, outcome model. For improving clinical performance Donobedian also suggests a stepwise approach as described in Box 3.1.

DOI 10.1007/978-90-481-2446-6_3,

Table 3.1 Definitions of structure, process, and outcome, adapted from Donobedian (2003)

Structure →	Process →	Outcome
1. Material resources; facilities and equipment (drugs, laboratory data etc.). 2. Human resources; number, variety, qualifications of professional and support personnel) 3. Organisational activities; teaching and research, supervision and performance review.	Activities; diagnosis, treatment, rehabilitation, prevention, and patient education- usually carried out by professional personnel, but also including others such as patient and their family	Changes in individuals and populations including; 1. Changes in health status, knowledge, and behaviour. 2. Satisfaction. Focusing on the patient and their family members.

Box 3.1 Steps for improving clinical performance

1. Determine what to monitor
2. Determine priorities in monitoring
3. Selecting an approach (es) for assessment of performance
4. Formulating criteria and standards
5. Obtaining the necessary information
6. Choosing when to monitor
7. Choosing how to monitor
8. Constructing a monitoring system
9. Bringing about the behaviour change

For improved quality of care in the elderly we must first define and measure the problem and the magnitude of the problem. We must also prioritise between problems and select the most important issue. Of course the aim must be improvement for the individual patient. But since quality in healthcare normally is complicated and multifactorial a systematic change in structures and processes is required.

3.2 Patient Benefit and -Risks

The so-called Hippocratic injunction states "Primum est non nocere", above all, do no harm. Is this really always the first aim? In helping a patient there is always a risk, but if a treatment is of no benefit it should not be used. How can we know if a treatment is of benefit for all patients, for a certain population, or for an individual patient? How can we get information, can we trust the authorities, the drug companies and the salesmen?

Before testing we can never know if a treatment is of benefit for a patient, even if there are scientific evidences for the population (see EBM below), so it is actually a trial. To do more good than harm we must first think of the consequences and with the patient discuss benefits and risk based on the questions in Box 3.2.

Box 3.2 Benefits and risks in treatment of an individual patient

How big is the problem for the patient?
Can we decrease the symptoms, cure or prevent disease or complications?
What is the evidence for the population and for the patient?
How big are the possible benefits, and the risks?
In a short- and long term perspective.

As health-care professionals we need to identify and solve the problem together with the patient, and we need to do it in a rational and cost-effective way. For a practitioner this is not easy based on the rapidly expanding progress within the medical area, increasing demand from patients, and the manipulation of information from various interests in the field. First we need drugs and other treatments with documented effects (efficacy) in the elderly. Then we need to select the most appropriate drug for the individual patient. The latter is complicated and evidence-based medicine (EBM) has been suggested as the method. Finally we need to communicate with the patient and establish a partnership (concordance).

3.3 Efficacy of (New) Drugs in the Elderly

Independent authority evaluation of drugs before market authorisation started in the 1930s in the United States after a tragic mistake in the formulation of a children syrup. In Japan the evaluations started in the 1950s and in many countries in Europe the trigger was the thalidomide tragedy of the 1960s which caused more than 10,000 malformed children.With the globalisation, rising cost in health care, escalation of the research and development cost, and the need for more effective and safe drugs there was a need for international harmonisation. ICH (International Conference of Harmonisation) was conceived in 1989 (ICH 2008).

3.3.1 International Harmonisation on Registration of New Drugs

The main feature of the harmonisation is guidelines and Common Technical Documents (CTD). The CTD gives a harmonised format and content for new product applications and in 2003 there was an agreement on implementation, in USA, Europe and Japan.

The ICH Topics are divided into four major categories.

- Organisation
- Quality—Chemical and pharmaceutical quality assurance (stability, impurities etc.)

- Safety—In vitro and in vivo pre-clinical studies (carcinogenicity, genotoxicity etc.)
- Efficacy—Clinical studies in human subject (dose response, carcinogenicity, Good Clinical Practices, Clinical Safety Data Management)

3.3.2 Requirements for Documentation and Use in the Elderly

The efficacy document E7 (ICH 1993) states that the drug should be studied in all patient groups, elderly included, for which they have a significant utility. It also includes new uses, new formulations and new combinations of established medicinal products when there is specific reason to expect that conditions common in the elderly (e.g. renal or hepatic impairment, impaired cardiac function, concomitant illness or medication) are likely to be encountered. This also applies for when the geriatric patients′ response (safety, tolerability, efficacy) is different from the non-geriatrics′.

The geriatric population comprises patients aged 65 years or more, but it is stated that it is important to seek patients in the older age range, 75 and older. The older the population likely to be users, the more important it is to include the very old. Geriatric patients should be included in meaningful numbers to permit comparisons of drug response to the younger group, at least 100 patients. For diseases associated with aging (e.g. Alzheimer) the majority of patients should be elderly. Clinical data should also be analysed and compared to seek age-related differences in adverse event rates, in effectiveness, and in dose response. If important differences are shown further evaluation is needed.

If used in the elderly, drug-drug interaction studies should be considered for digoxin and oral anticoagulants. For drugs that undergo extensive hepatic metabolism, effects of inducers (e.g. phenobarbital) and inhibitors (e.g. cimetidine) should be determined. For drugs metabolised by cytochrome P-450 enzymes it is critical to examine the effects of known inhibitors. Interaction studies with other drugs that are likely to be used with the test drug is also recommended.

3.4 Evidence Based Medicine

3.4.1 What EBM Is

Evidence Based Medicine (EBM) is the conscientious, explicit and judicious use of current best evidence in making decisions about the care of individual patients (Sackett et al. 1996). It combines and integrates clinical knowledge of the patient, with best available external clinical evidence from systematic research.

By best research evidence Sackett means clinically relevant research, often from the basic sciences of medicine, but especially from patient centred clinical research into the accuracy and precision of diagnostic tests (including the clinical examination), the power of prognostic markers, and the efficacy and safety of therapeutic, rehabilitative, and preventive regimens. New external clinical evidence both invalidates previously accepted diagnostic tests and treatments and replaces them with new ones that are more powerful, more accurate, more efficacious, and safer.

EBM is not "cook-book" medicine, it is not a way to cut costs in the short perspective, and it is not restricted to randomised trials and meta-analyses. Instead it focuses on a systematic approach to improve an individual patients care, for professional development and life long learning.

For more background, teaching and help on the practice of EBM the database at the Centre for Evidence Based Medicine (CEBM 2008) can be of help.

3.4.2 *Practising EBM*

A practitioner needs a systematic view to give his patient good quality care. It should start early in education and practice and be developed systematically over time. The basis for this view must be based on EBM. In Box 3.3 a theoretical model for practicing EBM is described (Sackett et al. 1996).

Box 3.3 Theoretical model for practicing EBM

1. Convert the patient problem into an answerable question
2. Track down the best evidence with which to answer that question
3. Critically appraise that evidence for its validity (closeness to the truth), impact (size of the effect), and applicability (usefulness)
4. Integrate the critical appraisal with your clinical expertise and with your patient's unique biology, values and circumstances
5. Evaluate your performance

Calculating the effect size of a therapeutic intervention is central (step 3 in Box 3.3). Different ways to calculate effects sizes can be applied as described in Table 3.2. All statements in this box actually describe the effect sizes correctly. Is the efficacy higher for drug A than for drug B? Probably not since the relative risk reduction is not identical. Instead the result probably reflects other differences such as higher morbidity (blood pressure, other risk factors, or diseases) in case A.

3.4.3 *Grading Evidences and Clinical Recommendations*

As described previously a central component in EBM is comparisons of interventions including step 2 (searching) and 3 (critically appraising) in Box 3.3. This can be very time-consuming. For help sources that have already undergone rigorous critical appraisal can be of very much help. Examples of this are found in Box 3.4.

Table 3.2 Effect size calculation and corresponding nomenclature based on two cases

Case A. In a clinical trial 1000 patients with hypertension were treated with drug A and 1000 patients with placebo. After one year there were 50 deaths in the drug A group and 100 deaths in the placebo group.

Statement	Term	Calculation
Reduced mortality by 50%	Relative risk reduction	From 100 to 50 deaths
Absolute reduced mortality by 5%	Absolute risk reduction	10% (100 of 1000 patients died) in placebo and 5% (50 of 1000) in drug A group.
Increased patient survival from 10% to 5%	Absolute risk reduction	From 10% to 5%
20 patients need to be treated to avoid one death.	Numbers needed to treat (NNT)	For 1000 patients 50 deaths were avoided (100 deaths in placebo and 50 in drug A group). 1000/50=100/5=20/1=20

Case B. In a clinical trial 1000 patients with hypertension were treated with drug B and 1000 patients with placebo. After one year there were 5 deaths in the drug B group and 10 deaths in the placebo group.

Statement	*Term*	*Calculation*
Reduced mortality by 50%	Relative risk reduction	From 10 to 5 deaths
Absolute reduced mortality by 0.5%	Absolute risk reduction	1% (10 of 1000 patients died) in placebo and 0.5% (5 of 1000) in drug B group.
Increased patient survival from 1% to 0.5%	Absolute risk reduction	From 1% to 0.5%
200 patients need to be treated to avoid one death.	Numbers needed to treat (NNT)	For 1000 patients 5 deaths were avoided (10 deaths in placebo and 5 in drug B group). 1000/5=100/0.5=200/1=200

Box 3.4 Examples of databases for evidence based reviews, clinical practice guidelines and recommendations

National Institute of Clinical Excellence (www.nice.org.uk/guidance)
Cochrane Reviews Database (www.cochrane.org/reviews)
UpToDate (www.uptodateinc.com/home/index.html)
Trip Database (http://www.tripdatabase.com/index.html)

Assessing methodological quality for each intervention, and grading the evidences based on the cumulated evidences and in comparison to other interventions is crucial for EBM. It is important to know how much we can trust the recommendations and clinical practice guidelines. Clinical guidelines are only as good as the evidence and judgments they are based on. A new system for grading the quality of evidence and the strength of recommendations have recently been developed (GRADE 2004). The aim is to make it easier for users to assess the judgments behind recommendations. Judgments about the strength of a recommendation require consideration of the balance between benefits and harms, the quality of the evidence, translation of the evidence into specific circumstances, and the certainty of the baseline risk. Finally it is also important to consider costs and resources before making a recommendation.

Based on four key elements (study design, study quality, consistency and directness) the system grades the evidences for each main outcome into four categories (high, moderate, low and very low) dependent on the quality of the evidences. Limitations in study quality, important inconsistency of results, or uncertainty about the directness of the evidence can lower the grade of evidence. Essentials in process, criteria and grading in the GRADE system is presented in Box 3.5.

Box 3.5 Essentials in process, criteria and grading in the GRADE system (GRADE 2004)

Sequential process for developing guidelines

First steps

1. Establishing the process—For example, prioritising problems, selecting a panel, declaring conflicts of interest, and agreeing on group processes

Preparatory steps

2. Systematic review—The first step is to identify and critically appraise or prepare systematic reviews of the best available evidence for all important outcomes
3. Prepare evidence profile for important outcomes—Profiles are needed for each subpopulation or risk group, based on the results of systematic reviews, and should include a quality assessment and a summary of findings

Grading quality of evidence and strength of recommendations

4. Quality of evidence for each outcome—Judged on information summarised in the evidence profile and based on the criteria described below
5. Relative importance of outcomes—Only important outcomes should be included in evidence profiles. The included outcomes should be classified as critical or important (but not critical) to a decision
6. Overall quality of evidence—The overall quality of evidence should be judged across outcomes based on the lowest quality of evidence for any of the critical outcomes.

7. Balance of benefits and harms—The balance of benefits and harms should be classified as net benefits, trade-offs, uncertain trade-offs, or no net benefits based on the important health benefits and harms
8. Balance of net benefits and costs—Are incremental health benefits worth the costs? Because resources are always limited, it is important to consider costs (resource utilisation) when making a recommendation
9. Strength of recommendation—Recommendations should be formulated to reflect their strength—that is, the extent to which one can be confident that adherence will do more good than harm

Subsequent steps

10. Implementation and evaluation—For example, using effective implementation strategies that address barriers to change, evaluation of implementation, and keeping up to date

Criteria for assigning grade of evidence for each outcome (step 4 above)
Type of evidence

- Randomised trial = high
- Observational study = low
- Any other evidence = very low

Decrease grade if:

- Serious (–1) or very serious (–2) limitation to study quality
- Important inconsistency (–1)
- Some (–1) or major (–2) uncertainty about directness
- Imprecise or sparse data (–1)
- High probability of reporting bias (–1)

Increase grade if:

- Strong evidence of association—significant relative risk of > 2 (< 0.5) based on consistent evidence from two or more observational studies, with no plausible confounders (+1)
- Very strong evidence of association—significant relative risk of > 5 (< 0.2) based on direct evidence with no major threats to validity (+2)
- Evidence of a dose response gradient (+1)
- All plausible confounders would have reduced the effect (+1)

Grading of the quality of evidences

- High = Further research is very unlikely to change our confidence in the estimate of effect.
- Moderate = Further research is likely to have an important impact on our confidence in the estimate of effect and may change the estimate.
- Low = Further research is very likely to have an important impact on our confidence in the estimate of effect and is likely to change the estimate.
- Very low = Any estimate of effect is very uncertain.

3.5 Shortcomings for EBM in the Elderly

3.5.1 General Aspects

Elderly are often high health-care consumers. They often have multiple diseases and use many drugs. Most old drugs but also relatively new ones have not documented clinical benefits in this group despite ICH guidelines presented above. Therefore the clinical skill of the practitioner is even more important as a basis for EBM. This includes not only the selection and information of a suitable medication and strategy for treatment but also the follow-up of effects, documentation and communication of the activities. Based on this, organisational and professional shortcomings are also major obstacles for optimal pharmacotherapy as described below.

3.5.2 Documentation of Clinical Benefits

For new drugs the authorities need documentation of the effectiveness and safety in the population where it is supposed to be used. If not, the use will be restricted as described above. Despite this there is a great lack of good quality scientific studies on the effects of different treatments in the elderly, especially in the 75+ (SBU 2003). Also there are few systematic reviews published for example as protocol/review in the Cochrane Reviews Database (88 hits using the search word "elderly" in keyword/abstract/title, 2008-07-11). Still there is prescribing, often due to lack of other therapeutic alternatives, lack of knowledge among prescriber or misleading information in the marketing. A full review of the clinical documentation and benefits of all or groups of drugs are beyond the scoop of this book but some examples are highlighted in Table 3.3 and in Box 3.6. In other chapters some disease states, specific drug classes and problems are presented.

Table 3.3 Some examples of evidence based reviews in the elderly from the Cochrane Review Database

Title	Background	Authors' conclusions
Antipsychotic medication for elderly people with schizophrenia (Marriott et al. 2006)	A large and growing number of older people across the world suffer from schizophrenia. Recommendations for their treatment are largely based on data extrapolated from studies of the use of antipsychotic medications in younger populations. In addition most manufacturers of such medications recommend prescription of reduced doses to the elderly. The evidence base for these assumptions is unclear and raises obvious questions regarding the appropriateness of such prescribing practice.	Antipsychotics may be widely used in the treatment of elderly people with schizophrenia, however, based on this systematic review, there are little robust data available to guide the clinician with respect to the most appropriate drug to prescribe. Clearly reported large short, medium and long-term randomised controlled trials with participants, interventions and primary outcomes that are familiar to those wishing to help elderly people with schizophrenia are long overdue.
Vaccines for preventing influenza in the elderly (Rivetti et al. 2006)	Influenza vaccination of elderly individuals is recommended worldwide and has been targeted toward the elderly and those at serious risk of complications.	In long-term care facilities, where vaccination is most effective against complications, the aims of the vaccination campaign are fulfilled, at least in part. However, according to reliable evidence the usefulness of vaccines in the community is modest. The apparent high effectiveness of the vaccines in preventing death from all causes may reflect a baseline imbalance in health status and other systematic differences in the two groups of participants.

Box 3.6 Some examples of efficacy documentation in the elderly

Blood pressure lowering drugs reduce risk of stroke (and myocardial infarction and death) in middle aged patients and even better in the elderly (NNT 86 vs 29 over 5 years) (Pearce 1998). However in the elderly the dysfunction in the autoregulation of brain blood flow, salt and fluids, and increased sensitivity to adverse effects and symptoms may change the picture.

Lipid modifying drugs (statins) have shown secondary cardio-vascular preventive effects (myocardial infarction) in a very large number of patients. Only one study (Shepherd et al. 2002) has been conducted in the elderly and showed similar results. However there was a significant increased cancer risk (25%).

In Parkinson's disease very few studies focus on the elderly although Parkinson's disease is significantly age-related (SBU 2003). In the studies few patients suffers mental side effects of the drugs, while in clinical practice almost half of elderly patients suffers such problems. Since the studies do not include patients with co-morbidity it does not reflect the clinical situation. In heart failure modern treatment recommendations are based on studies were the average age of the patients are 60–65 years, most of which did not even include patients over 80 (SBU 2003).

3.6 Organisational and Professional Aspcts

In the Cochrane Review Database, there were 81 protocols/reviews on the topic "Effective practice and organisation of care" (verified 2008-11-11). None of those were specific targeted towards the care of the elderly. Especially for the elderly, there are several organisational and professional shortcomings for optimal pharmacotherapy and a systematic and holistic view is needed. If a patient gets all care during her life time from one practitioner the organisational shortcomings becomes less important. This is however not possible or preferential in the modern health care system. Instead professional shortcomings can add more problems to the organisational level, as described in Chapter 7. A professional role can of course also delete or minimize organisational shortcomings, but this is often time consuming and more and more complex.

It is important that all relevant information, communication and documentation are available for all practitioners involved in the care of the patient. The organisational aspect is to make this possible and easily usable for care. The professional aspect is to correctly use the system for input and output. This includes documentation and follow-up on aims, planning and all other relevant activities. The patient opinion and need must also be addressed and documented. Many of the problems have the potential to cause errors. This is described in Chapter 7 and also in other chapters. Here we focus on the basic organisational and professional features of the medication system in the elderly.

3.6.1 Resources, Priorities and Ethical Principles

With an older population, higher demand, increasing cost and limited resources we have problems to satisfy all needs and priorities. These priorities and decisions are hard to do for the practitioner in relation to the patient and to the society. Priorities should be based on the three ethical principles (human dignity, needs and solidarity, cost-effectiveness) described in Box 3.7. Greater needs (severe diseases and low quality of life) and the weakest people (i.e. the elderly) should have priorities. Cost-effectiveness principles should only be used when comparing treatment methods for the same disease.

Box 3.7 The three ethical principles (National centre for priority setting in health care 2008)

Human dignity principle: every individual should have equal value and equal rights of personal characteristics and functions in society
Needs and solidarity principle: resources should be committed to the people or activities having the greatest need
Cost-effectiveness principle: in choosing among activities or interventions, a reasonable relationship should be attained between costs and effects, measured as improvement in health and increased quality of life

Based on these principles the priorities could be made at different levels. This should be started at the highest level among politicians and others, with mutual, transparent, long lasting decisions. Of course this is problematic. With the three ethical principles in mind we must all think of what we can do with limited resources and make our own priorities. EBM principles and methods as described above should be used. Some factors that increase the health-care costs are presented in Box 3.8, and should be considered. Several of the solutions presented in this and other chapters can be used.

Box 3.8 Factors that can increase costs in health-care

- New and expensive technologies and drugs can be interesting for practitioners despite low or now evidences for improved benefit/harm ratio
- Simple methods, often with proven benefits are forgotten such as; stop smoking, lower weight, reduce sleeping problems, sour throat and constipation etcetera
- Marketing
  - Broadened indications. Risk factors are launched as disease states that need treatment
  - Slide in indications. Similar disease states are treated despite low or no evidences
  - Ineffective methods. Irrational and selected argument that not gives the total picture
- The technological possible becomes the aim
- Increased expectations. It is not normal to get old, a struggle for "perfect" health
- Not used, incorrect used, and wasted medications

3.6.2 Patient Chart Order System

Traditionally different paper patient chart order systems have been used for documentation of all activities planned and performed. For each patient this could be hundreds and sometimes thousands of papers sorted by care occasion for each level of care. Also the documentation is sometimes incomplete and historical events and circumstances are hard to find. Recently some aspects of patient care such as laboratory lists and other tests and results have been included in electronic systems. Since medication chart orders belong to the most complicated issues this is often the last to be integrated.

There is no world wide solution or intention to develop a mutual chart order system. Not even in different countries or regions, this work has enough priority. With the expansion of electronic development and interface solutions it is surprising that the potential patient safety and work load benefits is not more highlighted. In a Swedish study on a university hospital several of the problems in pharmacotherapy perceived by physicians and nurses were related to patient chart order sheets (Eriksson et al. 1999). Electronic systems fully integrated or readable between different systems has the potential to decreases some of the problems, but it is not the universal system for improvement. For real improvement the system must support the patient care-system with documentation and easy access to objectives for treatment (including patient objectives), plan and results. It must also include prescribing support in the selection of medication (based on EBM in the elderly) and tools for follow up on patient outcomes or surrogate outcomes. Special emphasis should be put on errors in the medication reconciliation process. Experiences and improvements in the process as described below must be recognised in the development of future patient chart order systems

3.6.3 Prescribing

Traditionally drug prescriptions, hand written on paper, are a source for all types of errors. Use of computerised order entry (COE) and clinical decision support (CDS) tools can prevent serious medication errors (Leapfrog Group 2004). However new source for errors can occur based on errors in the system or by the prescriber. There is a great need for better COE/CDS especially in the treatment of the elderly. Drug-drug, drug-food, and disease-drug interactions, inappropriate drugs, and systematic help to follow up on activities and results, and also support in the prescriber-patient communication is needed. COE is one of the patient safety standards established and promoted by The Leapfrog Group based on the Institute of Medicine report, To Err Is Human (Chapter 7). A guide has been produced including three reports; an initial report, a report of costs, benefits and challenges, and a report on lessons from the field (Leapfrog 2004). The focus is also on CDS tools. CDS tools are just one of many important factors to consider in selecting a solution for improved prescribing. The purpose of the report is to help hospitals understand what vendors are in the COE marketplace. This information could be useful to hospitals as they start a search for a COE solution. It in no way covers the necessary detail to substitute for a careful exploration of a hospital's environment, objectives, available software, and the experience of other hospitals who have implemented these solutions.

Educational outreach can be a way for improvement. In a Cochrane review on educational outreach visits the authors concluded that alone or when combined with other interventions it have effects on prescribing that are relatively consistent and small, but potentially important (O'Brien et al. 2007). Their effects on other types of professional performance vary from small to modest improvements, and it is not possible from this review to explain that variation. We have shown positive effects after educational outreach visits to GP practices targeted at improving prescribing of some specific inappropriate drugs in the elderly. There were significant decreases in the active group compared to control group in prescribing of medium- and long-acting benzodiazepines and total benzodiazepines but not for antipsychotic drugs (Midlöv et al. 2006).

3.7 Conclusions

- Evidence based medicine combines and integrates clinical knowledge of the patient, with best available external clinical evidence from systematic research
- In the elderly evidence from systematic research is often lacking
- For quality of care in the elderly this put even higher emphasis on individualisation and on improving the structure and process of care delivery

References

CEBM (2008) Centre for Evidence Based Medicine. www.cebm.utoronto.ca/resources/cds.htm#be. Cited 30 Dec 2008

Donobedian A (2003) An introduction to quality assurance in health care. Oxford University Press, New York

Eriksson T, Henricson K, Arrhenius K, Höglund P, Stenberg P (1999) Perceived problems of pharmacotherapy. A problem detection study among physicians and nurses at a Swedish university hospital. Pharm World Sci 21: 190–193

GRADE (2004) Working Group. Grading quality of evidence and strength of recommendations. BMJ 328: 1490–1497

ICH (1993) Harmonised Tripartite Guideline (E7). Studies in support of special populations: Geriatrics. http://www.ich.org/LOB/media/MEDIA483.pdf. Cited 30 Dec 2008

ICH (2008) The International Conference on Harmonisation of Technical Requirements for Registration of Pharmaceuticals for Human Use. www.ich.org. Cited 30 Dec 2008

Leapfrog Group (2004) New guide for hospitals on computerised physician order entery (CPOE) gives hospitals much needed resource http://www.leapfroggroup.org/news/leapfrog_news/97902.Cited 30 Dec 2008

Marriott RG, Neil W, Waddingham S (2006) Antipsychotic medication for elderly people with schizophrenia. Cochrane Database of Systematic Reviews, Issue 1. Art. No.: CD005580. DOI:10.1002/14651858.CD005580

Midlöv P, Bondesson Å, Eriksson T, Nerbrand C, Höglund P (2006) Effects of educational outreach visits on prescribing of benzodiazepines and antipsychotic drugs to elderly patients in primary health care in southern Sweden. Family Practice 23: 60–64

O'Brien MA, Rogers S, Jamtvedt G, Oxman AD, Odgaard-Jensen J, Kristoffersen DT, Forsetlund L, Bainbridge D, Freemantle N, Davis DA, Haynes RB, Harvey EL (2007) Educational outreach visits: effects on professional practice and health care outcomes. Cochrane Database of Systematic Reviews Issue 4. Art. No.CD000409. DOI10.1002/14651858.CD000409.pub2

Pearce KA, Furberg CD, Psaty BM, Kirk J (1998) Cost-minimization and the number needed to treat in uncomplicated hypertension. Am J Hypertens11: 618–629

National centre for priority setting in health care (2008) Resolving health cares difficult choices-Survey of priority setting in sweden and an analysis of principles and guidelines on priorities in health care http://e.lio.se/prioriteringscentrum/Engelskversion/Engelska%20rapporter%20hela/2008.2.pdf. Cited 30 Dec 2008

Rivetti D, Jefferson T, Thomas R, Rudin M, Rivetti A, Di Pietrantonj C, Demicheli V (2006) Vaccines for preventing influenza in the elderly. Cochrane Database of Systematic Reviews Issue 3. Art. No CD004876. DOI 10.1002/14651858.CD004876.pub2

SBU (2003) The swedish council of on technology assessment in health care (SBU). Geriatric care and treatment. A systematic compilation of existing scientific literature. http://www.sbu.se/upload/Publikationer/Content1/2/Geriatric_Care/Geriatric_Care%20_Treatment.pdf. Cited 30 Dec 2008

Sackett DL, Rosenberg WM, Gray JA, Haynes RB, Richardson WS (1996) Evidence based medicine: what it is and what it isn't. BMJ 312: 71–72

Shepherd J, Blauw GJ, Murphy MB, Bollen EL, Buckley BM, Cobbe SM, Ford I (2002) Prospective study of pravastatin in the elderly at risk (PROSPER). Lancet 360: 1623–1630

Chapter 4
Inappropriate Drugs in the Elderly

Abstract Use of inappropriate drugs is common among elderly. These drugs are associated with an increased risk of adverse drug reactions in older adults. Here we focus on four groups of drugs that are frequently used by older patients but should, if possible, be avoided. These groups are: benzodiazepines, antipsychotic drugs, drugs with anticholinergic effects, and non-steroidal anti-inflammatory drugs (NSAID). Benzodiazepines, anticholinergic drugs and antipsychotic drugs may cause delirium, especially in the elderly. Possible severe adverse effects from NSAIDs are e.g. gastrointestinal bleeding, renal, and heart failure. Elderly patients are more susceptible to adverse drug reactions from all these drugs due to pharmacokinetical and pharmacodynamical alterations. In most cases there are safer alternatives.

Keywords Inappropriate drugs · Beer's criteria · Antipsychotics · Benzodiazepines · Anticholinergic drugs · NSAID

4.1 Introduction

Most drugs are appropriate also for elderly patients, at least when used in adequate dose, for the correct diagnosis and time period. Elderly are however more susceptible to adverse effects of drugs and therefore some drugs are inappropriate for the elderly. Inappropriate prescribing can be defined as prescribing that does not agree with accepted medical standards (Hanlon et al. 2001). Prescribing of inappropriate medications to elderly is common both in North America and Europe (Gallagher et al. 2007). Recommendations about the use or rather non-use have been made in different countries. There are several different criteria that describe medications deemed as inappropriate to elderly. In many scientific studies, medications are deemed as inappropriate to the elderly according to Beer's criteria. Beer's criteria were originally criteria for inappropriate medication use in nursing home residents. These criteria were developed to help assessing the quality of prescribing in elderly patients. Beer's criteria have been updated and are now applicable for all elderly patients (Fick et al. 2003). The criteria have been decided through a consensus panel with several experts and are applicable to elderly patients on a group

P. Midlöv et al., *Drug-Related Problems in the Elderly*,
DOI 10.1007/978-90-481-2446-6_4,

level. One should then also bare in mind that individual aspects have to be taken into account. Many drugs that are not included in Beer's criteria may be inappropriate for the individual older patient. To be useful to the clinician, these criteria have to be updated regularly.

There are other kinds of criteria that do not focus on specific medications but rather on the patient. One such example is Medication Appropriateness Index (MAI) with different questions as e.g. "Is there an indication for the drug?" (Samsa et al. 1994). This instrument may be more useful when assessing pharmacotherapy for the individual patient.

Inappropriate drug use is common among nursing home residents (Dhalla et al. 2002, Hagen et al. 2005) as well as in prescribing to elderly ambulatory care patients (Goulding 2004). Frail elderly that are most susceptible to adverse effects from drugs, use inappropriate drugs frequently and the use of these drugs is associated with impaired physical performance (Landi et al. 2007).

Having more than one prescriber increases the risk of inappropriate drug use (Piecoro et al. 2000, Dhalla et al. 2002). Thus, it is important that frail elderly have a physician that has knowledge of the patient's entire pharmacotherapy. It also emphasises the need for communication between different care givers.

In this chapter we focus on four different kinds of medications; benzodiazepines, antipsychotic drugs, drugs with anticholinergic effects, and non-steroidal anti-inflammatory drugs (NSAIDs). There are of course many other drugs that may be less appropriate in the elderly. There is e.g. an impairment of glucose counterregulation in the elderly, which explains the increased risk of hypoglycaemia caused by sulfonylureas in the elderly (Turnheim 1998). It is however impossible to include all drugs that might be inappropriate and we have focused on four groups of drugs that are frequently used among elderly.

Prevention is the most efficient way to minimise use of inappropriate medications among elderly. Reassessment of medication lists on a regular basis may be one way to both prevent and act on prevalent use of these medications.

4.2 Benzodiazepines

Benzodiazepines are widely used and their use is highest among the elderly (Flaherty 1998). According to Beer's criteria and different national recommendations, the use of long-acting benzodiazepines should be avoided in the elderly. Many physicians still prescribe benzodiazepines to elderly patients, contrary to official guidelines (Taylor et al. 1998). Approved indications for the use of benzodiazepines are the same for elderly patients as for younger adults. Anxiety and insomnia are the most common indications. Benzodiazepines remain common despite the development of newer drugs with less addictive potential. Selective serotonin re-uptake inhibitors (SSRI) for example are the first-line treatment for generalised anxiety disorder (Baldwin and Polkinghorn 2005). Benzodiazepines are also prescribed for multiple concomitant physical and psychological problems (Bogunovic and Greenfield 2004). There is not much scientific evidence that supports such prescribing.

4.2.1 Pharmacology

Many different physiological alterations make elderly more susceptible to benzodiazepines. Benzodiazepines are more likely to accumulate in the elderly due to alterations in pharmacokinetics. These alterations are not only due to drug distribution but also decreased metabolism (Sonne et al. 1991). The half-life of diazepam may increase fourfold between age 20 and 80 (Klotz et al. 1975). Alterations in pharmacodynamics can be even more important in explaining the altered response to benzodiazepines (Bogunovic and Greenfield 2004). Age-dependent changes in GABA-receptors may be responsible for the sensitivity of elderly to benzodiazepines (Klotz 1998). The aging brain has an increased sensitivity to the action of benzodiazepines. In one study the effects of a single dose of nitrazepam were compared with placebo in old and young adults. Despite similar plasma concentrations of nitrazepam, older persons made more mistakes in the psychomotor tests than younger persons (Castleden et al. 1977).

4.2.2 Risks

The consequences of benzodiazepine use in the elderly may be severe. Benzodiazepines are common in drug poisoning suicides in the elderly (Carlsten et al. 2003). This is especially apparent for the hypnotics; flunitrazepam and nitrazepam. Benzodiazepines are also associated with an increased risk of motor vehicle crashes in the elderly (Hebert et al. 2007).

Impairment of memory, delirium and immobility are some of the adverse drug reactions from benzodiazepines. Elderly patients in nursing homes often receive benzodiazepines inappropriately (Oborne et al. 2003). The frailest elderly, who are most susceptible to ADR from benzodiazepines, use these drugs and often for long term. In a Japanese study it was shown that benzodiazepines were prescribed for longer terms as patient age increased (Nomura et al. 2007). Sometimes elderly patients in nursing homes are treated with benzodiazepines without actually talking to their nurse or physician (Holmquist et al. 2005). This makes it hard evaluate the treatment.

Reducing benzodiazepine use in elderly patients is important for several reasons. Long-term use of benzodiazepines can accelerate cognitive decline in elderly patients (Paterniti et al. 2002). The elderly experience excessive sedation from benzodiazepines compared with younger individuals (Lechin et al. 1996). Benzodiazepine use by elderly patients are not only associated with cognitive side effects

(Lechin et al. 1996, Gray et al. 1999), but also increases the risk of falls and hip fractures (Passaro et al. 2000, Ray et al. 2000, Wang et al. 2001). Daily dose and longer duration of benzodiazepine use is associated with higher risk of fracture (van der Hooft et al. 2008). These fractures lead to great hospitalisation costs. In a European study it was estimated that costs of accidental injuries related to benzodiazepine use in the EU are between Euro 1.5 and Euro 2.2 billion each year. More than 90% of these costs were in the elderly with fractures as the major contributor (Panneman et al. 2003).

4.2.3 Insomnia

Sleep disturbances are common in the elderly. These disturbances are often secondary to medical illness and/or medication use (Martin et al. 2000). Illnesses could be anxiety disorders or any illness that may disturb sleep due to pain or nocturia. Medications that may cause sleep disturbances are e.g. beta-blockers, corticosteroids and SSRIs. If the sleep disturbance is secondary the treatment should be focused on the underlying cause. If there is no such cause the sleep disturbance is said to be primary. First-line treatment should then be improvement of sleep hygiene (Box 4.1).

Box 4.1 Improving sleep hygiene

Dark and quiet bedroom
Avoid evening use of stimulating agents, e.g. alcohol or caffeine
Avoid day-time naps
Avoid medications that may cause sleep disturbance
Optimise treatment of conditions that may contribute to insomnia

Before initiating any pharmacotherapy the patient should be asked about sleep-wake patterns, napping etc. Disturbed sleep is common among elderly (Vitiello 1997). In a study on persons 81 years or older, more than one third had problems with their sleep (Giron et al. 2002). There are better tolerated pharmacological alternatives than benzodiazepines (Hemmeter et al. 2000) and many times identifying problems that cause the sleep disturbance may solve the problem.

When non-pharmacological treatment is not sufficient benzodiazepines have been first-line treatment. There are however several disadvantages, besides the general adverse effects, benzodiazepines may affect sleep architecture and worsening sleep apnoea. Long-acting benzodiazepines have high risk of daytime sedation in older adults (Bachman 1992). Sleep-wake pattern may then be disturbed. Instead of benzodiazepines zopiclone or zolpidem are preferred when pharmacotherapy is needed. These drugs have fewer side effects and less risk of dependence compared with benzodiazepines (Schneider 2002).

4.2.4 Use and Discontinuation

The use of benzodiazepines should be avoided. There are other safer pharmacological alternatives. Benzodiazepine withdrawal may play a role in the occurrence of delirium in the elderly. Other withdrawal symptoms include tremor, agitation, insomnia and seizures (Turnheim 2003). Thus, when there is long-term use of benzodiazepines abrupt discontinuation might be difficult. Discontinuation should however not be withheld but done slowly and step-wise. If benzodiazepines are used in the elderly, short-acting benzodiazepines such as oxazepam are preferred, because they do not accumulate in the elderly to the same extent (Kompoliti and Goetz 1998). If short-acting benzodiazepines are used they should be prescribed with caution, at low doses, and for short periods. As with all pharmacotherapy the effects should be evaluated. Benzodiazepines are sometimes used as a behavioural control. One should always ask if this use is for the benefit of staff or the benefit of the patient. The presence of staff may be sufficient for behavioural control.

4.3 Antipsychotic Drugs

Antipsychotic drugs are associated with high risk of unwanted effects in the elderly. Serious adverse events occur frequently within the first month of initiating antipsychotic therapy in elderly with dementia (Rochon et al. 2008). There is an increased risk of well-known adverse effects as tardive dyskinesia and parkinsonism (Avorn et al. 1995, Woerner et al. 1998). Tardive dyskinesia, or involuntary movements, is very unpleasant and troublesome to the elderly patient. The risk of tardive dyskinesia in older patients is high even with relatively short treatment with low doses (Jeste et al. 1999). Other adverse effects e.g. worsening cognitive decline are also more frequent in the elderly (McShane et al. 1997). Most of these drugs are not well-studied for other diagnoses than psychotic diseases. In treatment of dementia, the efficacy of antipsychotic drugs is low, and the efficacy rate is equivalent to the side effect rate (Lanctot et al. 1998). Despite these facts antipsychotic drugs are often used in elderly without a psychotic disorder. In a British audit-study in primary care, it was found that the use of antipsychotic drugs was infrequent, but most was unsatisfactory (Mortimer et al. 2005). The lack of psychotic disorder diagnosis among the users of these drugs was common. There is often no documentation of indications and evaluations when elderly are treated with antipsychotic drugs (Holmquist et al. 2003). Considering the high risk of ADR, this is unsatisfactory. Antipsychotic drugs as well as benzodiazepines are associated with an increased risk of falls (Landi et al. 2005). Several studies have confirmed that elderly patients in nursing homes or in their own homes are prescribed antipsychotic drugs without a correct indication (Golden et al. 1999, Ruths et al. 2001, Fahey et al. 2003, Hagen et al. 2005).

In a Norwegian study on nursing home residents clinically relevant medication problems were identified in 76% of the patients and antipsychotics were the class most often involved (Ruths et al. 2003). In an Australian study on nursing home residents the proportion of patients taking antipsychotics was 24% in 2003 and this was roughly the same as in 1993 (27%) and in 1998 (23%) (Snowdon et al. 2005). To reduce the use of antipsychotic drugs in the elderly is still an important issue. For many patients antipsychotic drugs can be withdrawn without detrimental effect on functional or cognitive status (Ballard et al. 2008). Even if there is no dependence as with benzodiazepines, abrupt discontinuation may be difficult. A stepwise approach is recommended. Newer antipsychotics are frequently used to treat behavioural symptoms in patients with dementia. They are sometimes referred to as atypical antipsychotic drugs. Atypical antipsychotics may achieve better control of psychotic symptoms in elderly (Brodaty et al. 2003). With risperidone elderly however achieve higher plasma concentrations than younger patients with similar dosage (Aichhorn et al. 2005). Low doses and thorough evaluation is important. In a recent study on patients with Alzheimer's disease there was an increased long-term risk of mortality in patients who were prescribed antipsychotic medication (Ballard et al. 2009). Antipsychotic drugs should, if at all, be prescribed cautiously in elderly.

4.4 NSAID

The function of the immune system is known to decline in the elderly. Autoimmune reactions and diseases increase with age although in general reactivity against antigens decrease (Wick and Grubeck-Loebenstein 1997). Non-steroidal anti-inflammatory drugs (NSAID) encompass several different substances, all with the ability to inhibit cyclooxygenase which is an enzyme used in the synthesis of prostaglandins. Prostaglandins mediate physiologic effects in several organs, such as maintain renal blood flow and glomerular filtration. When such a physiologic effect is suppressed by NSAIDs, impairment in renal function may result. Another example is that prostaglandins are important to protect the mucosa of the stomach and duodenum. Removal of this protection may result in peptic ulcers. There is an increased risk of gastrointestinal bleeding from NSAID with old age (Hernandez-Diaz and Rodriguez 2000). Non-steroidal anti-inflammatory drugs are also associated with gastric ulcers (Garcia Rodriguez and Hernandez-Diaz 2004). The frequency of ADR caused by NSAID increases with age (Wolfe et al. 1999). Use of NSAID is quite common in all age groups. The symptoms of these ADR may initially be vague as e.g. tiredness. This could then be the only symptom of anaemia due to gastrointestinal bleeding. Heart failure due to NSAID is another common ADR (Huerta et al. 2006). Non-steroidal anti-inflammatory drugs are associated with an increased risk for heart failure (Garcia Rodriguez and Hernandez-Diaz 2003, Huerta et al. 2006).Heart failure is a common reason for hospitalisation in the elderly (Shahar et al. 2004). Patients with renal failure, diabetes or hypertension are at greater risk of developing heart failure when taking NSAIDs (Garcia Rodriguez and Hernandez-Diaz 2003). The use of NSAID in the elderly is thus associated with high risk of severe ADR.

4.5 Drugs with Anticholinergic Effects

Anticholinergic drug use is common among elderly (Ness et al. 2006). Acetylcholine is a neurotransmitter that is present in several parts of the brain. It has mainly excitatory effects. There are two important groups of acetylcholine receptors in the brain; nicotinic and muscarinic. Drugs that block muscarinic receptors are used e.g. in treatment of Parkinson's disease. Elderly patients are more susceptible to anticholinergic effects. Serum anticholinergic activity (SAA) can be detected in most older persons and even low SAA is associated with cognitive impairment (Mulsant et al. 2003). Elderly patients taking anticholinergic drugs are more likely to be mildly cognitively impaired and have an increased risk of delirium (Lechevallier-Michel et al. 2005, Ancelin et al. 2006). It has been shown that elderly are more susceptible to cognitive impairment due to anticholinergic drugs than younger adults (Naranjo et al. 2000). Anticholinergic effects include tachycardia, urinary retention, constipation, dry mouth, blurred vision and delirium. These are common symptoms in elderly patients and it is important to have anticholinergic effects of drugs in mind in these cases.

A wide variety of drugs have anticholinergic effects, e.g. antipsychotic drugs, urology drugs, anti-parkinsonian drugs and antidepressants (Table 4.1). Many other drugs may have little anticholinergic effects. Although one such medication may not result in anticholinergic effects, the concurrent use of several medications may result in anticholinergic effects (Mulsant et al. 2003). Whenever an elderly patient present with cognitive impairment, consideration should be given to withdraw or at least lower the dose of such drugs. This has to be done before considering adding drugs.

Tricyclic antidepressants have anticholinergic side effects that are augmented in the elderly. Anticholinergic symptoms are clinically meaningful to elderly patients (Ness et al. 2006). All treatment with drugs with known anticholinergic effects should be thoroughly evaluated and whenever possible in the elderly withdrawn or replaced with other drugs.

Table 4.1 Anticholinergic drugs, some examples

Drug	Use	ATC*
Amitryptiline	Depression	N06A A09
Atropine	Spasmolytic	A03B A01
Diphenhydramine	Antihistaminic	R05C A10
Disopyramide	Antiarrhytmic	C01B A03
Hydroxyzine	Sedating	N05B B01
Hyoscyamine	Spasmolytic	A03B A03
Orphenadrine	Parkinson's disease	M03B C01
Oxybutynin	Spasmolytic	G04B D04
Scopolamine	Spasmolytic	A04A D01

*ATC therapeutic group based on the World Health Organisation Nordic Anatomical Therapeutic Chemical Classification Index (ATC) codes.

4.6 Conclusions

- Use of inappropriate drugs is common among elderly
- Benzodiazepines are addictive and associated with high risk of adverse effects
- Antipsychotic drugs are often used in the elderly without any psychotic disorder
- Benzodiazepines and antipsychotic drugs are associated with cognitive impairment and increased risk of falls
- Non-steroidal anti-inflammatory drugs are associated with severe adverse drug reactions e.g. heart failure and gastrointestinal bleeding
- Drugs with anticholinergic effects may cause delirium but also tachycardia, urinary retention, constipation, dry mouth and blurred vision

References

Aichhorn W, Weiss U, Marksteiner J et al. (2005) Influence of age and gender on risperidone plasma concentrations. J Psychopharmacol 19(4): 395–401

Ancelin ML, Artero S, Portet F et al. (2006) Non-degenerative mild cognitive impairment in elderly people and use of anticholinergic drugs: longitudinal cohort study. BMJ 332: 455–459

Avorn J, Bohn RL, Mogun H et al. (1995) Neuroleptic drug exposure and treatment of parkinsonism in the elderly: a case-control study. Am J Med 99(1): 48–54

Bachman DL (1992) Sleep disorders with aging: evaluation and treatment. Geriatrics 47(9): 53–56, 59–61

Baldwin DS and Polkinghorn C (2005) Evidence-based pharmacotherapy of Generalized Anxiety Disorder. Int J Neuropsychopharmacol 8(2): 293–302

Ballard C, Hanney ML, Theodoulou M et al. (2009) The dementia antipsychotic withdrawal trial (DART-AD): long-term follow-up of a randomised placebo-controlled trial. The Lancet Neurology DOI:10.1016/S1474-4422(08)70295-3

Ballard C, Lana MM, Theodoulou M et al. (2008) A randomised, blinded, placebo-controlled trial in dementia patients continuing or stopping antipsychotics (the DART-AD trial). PLoS Med 5(4): e76

Bogunovic OJ and Greenfield SF (2004) Practical geriatrics: Use of benzodiazepines among elderly patients. Psychiatr Serv 55(3): 233–235

Brodaty H, Ames D, Snowdon J et al. (2003) A randomized placebo-controlled trial of risperidone for the treatment of aggression, agitation, and psychosis of dementia. J Clin Psychiatry 64(2): 134–143

Carlsten A, Waern M, Holmgren P et al. (2003) The role of benzodiazepines in elderly suicides. Scand J Public Health 31(3): 224–248

Castleden CM, George CF, Marcer D et al. (1977) Increased sensitivity to nitrazepam in old age. Br Med J 1(6052): 10–12

Dhalla IA, Anderson GM, Mamdani MM et al. (2002) Inappropriate prescribing before and after nursing home admission. J Am Geriatr Soc 50(6): 995–1000

Fahey T, Montgomery AA, Barnes J et al. (2003) Quality of care for elderly residents in nursing homes and elderly people living at home: controlled observational study. BMJ 326(7389): 580

Fick DM, Cooper JW, Wade WE et al. (2003) Updating the Beers criteria for potentially inappropriate medication use in older adults: results of a US consensus panel of experts. Arch Intern Med 163(22): 2716–2724

Flaherty JH (1998) Psychotherapeutic agents in older adults. Commonly prescribed and over- the-counter remedies: causes of confusion. Clin Geriatr Med 14(1): 101–127

Gallagher P, Barry P, O'Mahony D (2007) Inappropriate prescribing in the elderly. J Clin Pharm Ther 32(2): 113–121

Garcia Rodriguez LA and Hernandez-Diaz S (2003) Nonsteroidal antiinflammatory drugs as a trigger of clinical heart failure. Epidemiology 14(2): 240–246

Garcia Rodriguez LA and Hernandez-Diaz S (2004) Risk of uncomplicated peptic ulcer among users of aspirin and nonaspirin nonsteroidal antiinflammatory drugs. Am J Epidemiol 159(1): 23–31

Giron MS, Forsell Y, Bernsten C et al. (2002) Sleep problems in a very old population: drug use and clinical correlates. J Gerontol A Biol Sci Med Sci 57(4): M236–M240

Golden AG, Preston RA, Barnett SD et al. (1999) Inappropriate medication prescribing in homebound older adults. J Am Geriatr Soc 47(8): 948–953

Goulding MR (2004) Inappropriate medication prescribing for elderly ambulatory care patients. Arch Intern Med 164(3): 305–312

Gray SL, Lai KV, Larson EB (1999) Drug-induced cognition disorders in the elderly: incidence, prevention and management. Drug Saf 21(2): 101–122

Hagen BF, Armstrong-Esther C, Quail P et al. (2005) Neuroleptic and benzodiazepine use in long-term care in urban and rural Alberta: characteristics and results of an education intervention to ensure appropriate use. Int Psychogeriatr 17(4): 631–652

Hanlon JT, Schmader KE, Ruby CM et al. (2001) Suboptimal prescribing in older inpatients and outpatients. J Am Geriatr Soc 49(2): 200–209

Hebert C, Delaney JA, Hemmelgarn B et al. (2007) Benzodiazepines and elderly drivers: a comparison of pharmacoepidemiological study designs. Pharmacoepidemiol Drug Saf 16(8): 845–849

Hemmeter U, Muller M, Bischof R et al. (2000) Effect of zopiclone and temazepam on sleep EEG parameters, psychomotor and memory functions in healthy elderly volunteers. Psychopharmacology (Berl) 147(4): 384–396

Hernandez-Diaz S and Rodriguez LA (2000) Association between nonsteroidal anti-inflammatory drugs and upper gastrointestinal tract bleeding/perforation: an overview of epidemiologic studies published in the 1990s. Arch Intern Med 160(14): 2093–2099

Holmquist IB, Svensson B, Hoglund P (2003) Psychotropic drugs in nursing- and old-age homes: relationships between needs of care and mental health status. Eur J Clin Pharmacol 59(8–9): 669–676

Holmquist IB, Svensson B, Hoglund P (2005) Perceived anxiety, depression, and sleeping problems in relation to psychotropic drug use among elderly in assisted-living facilities. Eur J Clin Pharmacol 61(3): 215–224

Huerta C, Varas-Lorenzo C, Castellsague J et al. (2006) Non-steroidal anti-inflammatory drugs and risk of first hospital admission for heart failure in the general population. Heart 92(11): 1610–1615

Jeste DV, Lacro JP, Palmer B et al. (1999) Incidence of tardive dyskinesia in early stages of low-dose treatment with typical antipsychotics in older patients. Am J Psychiatry 156(2): 309–311

Klotz U (1998) Effect of age on pharmacokinetics and pharmacodynamics in man. Int J Clin Pharmacol Ther 36(11): 581–585

Klotz U, Avant GR, Hoyumpa A et al. (1975) The effects of age and liver disease on the disposition and elimination of diazepam in adult man. J Clin Invest 55(2): 347–359

Kompoliti K and Goetz CG (1998) Neuropharmacology in the elderly. Neurol Clin 16(3): 599–610

Lanctot KL, Best TS, Mittmann N et al. (1998) Efficacy and safety of antipsychotics in behavioral disorders associated with dementia. J Clin Psychiatry 59(10): 550–561

Landi F, Onder G, Cesari M et al. (2005) Psychotropic medications and risk for falls among community-dwelling frail older people: an observational study. J Gerontol A Biol Sci Med Sci 60(5): 622–626

Landi F, Russo A, Liperoti R et al. (2007) Impact of inappropriate drug use on physical performance among a frail elderly population living in the community. Eur J Clin Pharmacol 63(8): 791–799

Lechevallier-Michel N, Molimard M, Dartigues JF et al. (2005) Drugs with anticholinergic properties and cognitive performance in the elderly: results from the PAQUID Study. Br J Clin Pharmacol 59(2): 143–151

Lechin F, van der Dijs B, Benaim M (1996) Benzodiazepines: tolerability in elderly patients. Psychother Psychosom 65(4): 171–182

Martin J, Shochat T, Ancoli-Israel S (2000) Assessment and treatment of sleep disturbances in older adults. Clin Psychol Rev 20(6): 783–805

McShane R, Keene J, Gedling K et al. (1997) Do neuroleptic drugs hasten cognitive decline in dementia? Prospective study with necropsy follow up. BMJ 314(7076): 266–270

Mortimer AM, Shepherd CJ, Rymer M et al. (2005) Primary care use of antipsychotic drugs: an audit and intervention study. Ann Gen Psychiatry 4: 18 DOI:10.1186/1744-859X-4-18

Mulsant BH, Pollock BG, Kirshner M et al. (2003) Serum anticholinergic activity in a community-based sample of older adults: relationship with cognitive performance. Arch Gen Psychiatry 60(2): 198–203

Naranjo CA, Fourie J, Herrmann N et al. (2000) Probing peripheral and central cholinergic system responses. J Psychiatry Neurosci 25(4): 325–336

Ness J, Hoth A, Barnett MJ et al. (2006) Anticholinergic medications in community-dwelling older veterans: prevalence of anticholinergic symptoms, symptom burden, and adverse drug events. Am J Geriatr Pharmacother 4(1): 42–51

Nomura K, Nakao M, Sato M et al. (2007) The long-term prescription of benzodiazepines, psychotropic agents, to the elderly at a university hospital in Japan. Tohoku J Exp Med 212(3): 239–246

Oborne CA, Hooper R, Swift CG et al. (2003) Explicit, evidence-based criteria to assess the quality of prescribing to elderly nursing home residents. Age Ageing 32(1): 102–108

Panneman MJ, Goettsch WG, Kramarz P et al. (2003) The costs of benzodiazepine-associated hospital-treated fall Injuries in the EU: a Pharmo study. Drugs Aging 20(11): 833–839

Passaro A, Volpato S, Romagnoni F et al. (2000) Benzodiazepines with different half-life and falling in a hospitalized population: The GIFA study. Gruppo Italiano di Farmacovigilanza nell'Anziano. J Clin Epidemiol 53(12): 1222–1229

Paterniti S, Dufouil C, Alperovitch A (2002) Long-term benzodiazepine use and cognitive decline in the elderly: the Epidemiology of Vascular Aging Study. J Clin Psychopharmacol 22(3): 285–293

Piecoro LT, Browning SR, Prince TS et al. (2000) A database analysis of potentially inappropriate drug use in an elderly medicaid population. Pharmacotherapy 20(2): 221–228

Ray WA, Thapa PB, Gideon P (2000) Benzodiazepines and the risk of falls in nursing home residents. J Am Geriatr Soc 48(6): 682–685

Rochon PA, Normand SL, Gomes T et al. (2008) Antipsychotic therapy and short-term serious events in older adults with dementia. Arch Intern Med 168(10): 1090–1096

Ruths S, Straand J, Nygaard HA (2001) Psychotropic drug use in nursing homes – diagnostic indications and variations between institutions. Eur J Clin Pharmacol 57(6–7): 523–528

Ruths S, Straand J, Nygaard HA (2003) Multidisciplinary medication review in nursing home residents: what are the most significant drug-related problems? The Bergen District Nursing Home (BEDNURS) study. Qual Saf Health Care 12(3): 176–180

Samsa GP, Hanlon JT, Schmader KE et al. (1994) A summated score for the medication appropriateness index: development and assessment of clinimetric properties including content validity. J Clin Epidemiol 47(8): 891–896

Schneider DL (2002) Insomnia: Safe and effective therapy for sleep problems in the older patient. Geriatrics 57(5): 24–26

Shahar E, Lee S, Kim J et al. (2004) Hospitalized heart failure: rates and long-term mortality. J Card Fail 10(5): 374–379

Snowdon J, Day S, Baker W (2006) Current use of psychotropic medication in nursing homes. Int Psychogeriatr 18(2): 241–250

Sonne J, Loft S, Dossing M et al. (1991) Single dose pharmacokinetics and pharmacodynamics of oral oxazepam in very elderly institutionalised subjects. Br J Clin Pharmacol 31(6): 719–722

Taylor S, McCracken CF, Wilson KC et al. (1998) Extent and appropriateness of benzodiazepine use. Results from an elderly urban community. Br J Psychiatry 173: 433–438

Turnheim K (1998) Drug dosage in the elderly. Is it rational? Drugs Aging 13(5): 357–379
Turnheim K (2003) When drug therapy gets old: pharmacokinetics and pharmacodynamics in the elderly. Exp Gerontol 38(8): 843–853
van der Hooft CS, Schoofs MW, Ziere G et al. (2008) Inappropriate benzodiazepine use in older adults and the risk of fracture. Br J Clin Pharmacol 66(2): 276–282
Vitiello MV (1997) Sleep disorders and aging: understanding the causes. J Gerontol A Biol Sci Med Sci 52(4): M189–M191
Wang PS, Bohn RL, Glynn RJ et al. (2001) Hazardous benzodiazepine regimens in the elderly: effects of half-life, dosage, and duration on risk of hip fracture. Am J Psychiatry 158(6): 892–898
Wick G and Grubeck-Loebenstein B (1997) The aging immune system: primary and secondary alterations of immune reactivity in the elderly. Exp Gerontol 32(4–5): 401–413
Woerner MG, Alvir JM, Saltz BL et al. (1998) Prospective study of tardive dyskinesia in the elderly: rates and risk factors. Am J Psychiatry 155(11): 1521–1528
Wolfe MM, Lichtenstein DR, Singh G (1999) Gastrointestinal toxicity of nonsteroidal antiinflammatory drugs. N Engl J Med 340(24): 1888–1899

Chapter 5
Drugs and Common Health Conditions in Old Age

Abstract Elderly persons are often treated with pharmaceuticals for many different conditions, both for chronic diseases and common ailments in old age. Many prescribed medicines and herbal remedies as well as over the counter purchased drugs are frequently used in the older population. The resulting polypharmacy poses a challenge to physicians to master complicated pharmacological issues and combinations of drugs. Adverse drug effects and interactions between combinations of drugs essential for the medical treatment for chronic diseases such as high blood pressure, diabetes or osteoporosis, are some of the problems to be solved. Often the normal course of aging in the human body gives rise to ailments that should not really be treated with drugs at all. To "medicalise" aging, is to put our patients at risk in many potentially dangerous ways. Sometimes, in a long term perspective, the cure can be worse than the condition itself for the patient.

In this chapter common geriatric conditions will be described with special attention to the pharmacological treatment and hazards of drug treatment in the elderly. A number of frequently occurring complaints and ailments in the aging population will be described in connection with drug treatment. Gastrointestinal conditions such as constipation, peptic ulcers, gastritis and dryness of the mouth will be covered as well as kidney failure, urinary incontinence, osteoporosis, falls and fractures, sarcopenia, orthostatic hypotension and vertigo. These chosen examples are conditions that can be treated with, and often should be treated with, drugs. But what are the drawbacks to this?

Keywords Constipation · Peptic ulcers · Dryness of the mouth · Renal failure · Urinary incontinence · Osteoporosis · Sarcopenia · Orthostatic hypotension · Vertigo

5.1 Gastrointestinal Health Problems

There are many prevalent conditions in the elderly that can interfere with the normal pharmacokinetic process. The changes in the gastrointestinal tract due to aging do not normally give any problems with drug treatment but in combination with diverse chronic ailments, they do. The absorption of drugs can be disturbed by the

P. Midlöv et al., *Drug-Related Problems in the Elderly*,
DOI 10.1007/978-90-481-2446-6_5,

inability to properly swallow pills or capsules caused by dry mouth and sometimes a severely inflamed gastric mucosa can delay or inhibit drug absorption. Constipation is very often a problem connected with aging and can also interfere with the pharmacokinetic process in the elderly.

5.2 Constipation

As the human body gets older a slow decline in bowel movements occurs and this can create problems with constipation. The definition of constipation is less than three defecations a week and/or uncomfortable straining on defecation. There are no certain statistics of how high the prevalence of constipation is in the older population but as many as 25–30% could be afflicted by this common ailment (Talley et al. 1992). The use of laxatives increases with old age and is a sign of how frequent the problem is. In Swedish nursing homes as many as 70% are using laxatives more or less regularly (Kragh 2004).

There are two different mechanisms behind ordinary causes of constipation, functional and outlet obstructions. Functional constipation is caused by the slower movement of the colon, peristalsis, which comes with old age, often in combination with less physical activity and less intake of fibre containing food. Outlet obstruction is a result of incapacity to empty the rectum from faeces often due to too large masses of stool blocking the anus. It can also be caused by anal stricture from haemorrhoids or scar tissue caused by fissures.

Many diseases that can cause physical inactivity and decreased intake of fluids and food can have constipation as a common symptom. Acute infections with dehydration or chronic diseases as heart failure, diabetes, Parkinson's disease, obstructive pulmonary disease or terminal cancer, are some.

Among other risk factors for developing constipation are drugs. Certain drug classes are more known to cause constipation than others. Many different drugs can give rise to this side effect by diverse mechanisms such as to slow down colonic motility or lower the fluid contents of the stool. Both over-the-counter drugs and herbal remedies should be taken into consideration when examining and treating a patient with severe or chronic constipation (Box 5.1).

Box 5.1 Drugs that can cause constipation

Opioids
Calcium channel blockers
Anticholinergic drugs (e.g. tricyclic antidepressants, urological spasmolytics)
Iron supplements
Calcium supplements
Antacids (e.g. aluminium hydroxide)
Anti-inflammatory drugs
Chronic use of laxatives

Besides causing loss of appetite and quality of life, longstanding and severe constipation can lead to diverticulosis, diverticulitis and in worst cases perforation of the large intestine with life threatening peritonitis (McConnell et al. 2003). Diverticulosis, irritable bowel syndrome and haemorrhoids are caused by chronic constipation and can lead to bleeding and anaemia.

5.2.1 Treatment

Treatment options for constipation are actions directed at the underlying causes. Increasing the intake of fluids and fibres, to exercise regularly and in some cases, laxatives, are essential options (Tramonte et al. 1997). The risks of long term use of laxatives are low levels of potassium in the blood and injuries to the nerves and muscles of the colon causing dysmotility. In worse cases, irreversible damage to the colonic activity can occur and lead to so called "megacolon". Unfortunately, patients can then try to overcome the worsening constipation by increasing the laxative dosages and number of preparations being used. Stimulating laxatives can especially give rise to these complications. A number of drug classes can cause or worsen constipation, opioids, calcium channel blockers, anticholinergic medication, and supplements of calcium and iron (Box 5.1). In most cases prophylactic treatment with bulk laxatives, increased intake of fluids and fibres in combination with physical activity are enough to forestall constipation.

When prescribing strong opioids as analgesics for severe pain, it is even recommended to combine the treatment with prophylactic use of laxatives to avoid constipation. The effect of opioids on the bowel is to cause almost no movement at all in the bowels and therefore it is unavoidable to use stimulating laxatives sometimes combined with bulk forming preparations.

It is important to bear in mind that constipation is common in old age and often has negative effects on both health and quality of life. Constipation is often caused by chronic diseases and by many different drugs. It is best treated by life style changes and drugs that can cause constipation should be avoided or discontinued if possible.

5.3 Dryness of the Mouth

More than four hundred drugs are known to cause dryness of the mouth as an unwanted side-effect. Ten of the fifteen most used drugs among people over 65 can cause uncomfortable dryness of the mouth which the patients don't always associate with their medication (Thomson et al. 2000). According to Ship et al. 2002, as many as 30% of the population 65 years and older experience xerostomia.

Low secretion of saliva and less mucin in the produced saliva are not unusual in older individuals. Saliva has a number of protective functions of which the most important is protection against irritation by both chemical and mechanical trauma to the mucous membranes of the oral cavity. Saliva also facilitates the act of speaking and swallowing food and drink. It protects against caries by buffering and helping to remineralise tooth enamel. Saliva plays a very important role for enhancing the experience of taste and contains enzymes for the digestion of food. Signs of low secretion of saliva are dry fissured lips, red or fissured tongue as well as sore ulcers around the corners of the mouth.

A person can experience dryness of the mouth even though the major salivatory glands are functioning normally, the reason being that the small saliva producing glands situated in the membranes of the tongue cease to function. Other symptoms of mouth dryness besides the unpleasant sensation are redness of the mucous membranes in the oral cavity, dull lustreless membranes, widespread caries or bacterial and fungal infections.

Healthy aging includes a good nutritional status. To reach this, both the food contents and the ability to consume food in a proper way, are essential. With passing age, both the quality of the saliva and the mucous membranes deteriorates and swallowing often becomes more difficult. To chew and swallow properly is not always easy for an elderly individual due to dry mucous membranes in the mouth and pharynx, as well as malfunctioning dental prosthesis or no teeth at all. This problem is very common in old age (Turner and Ship 2007).

5.3.1 Risk Factors for Dryness of the Mouth

Besides drugs, other conditions that can lead to mouth dryness are radiation against the neck, fever, concomitant diseases such as rheumatoid arthritis and other connective tissue diseases (scleroderma, sicca syndrome), Parkinson's disease, numeral psychiatric conditions and stroke with paralysis, dysphagia, neglect or oral apraxia. Damage to the mouth can arise due to drug treatment through different mechanisms and here are some examples.

- Stomatitis: NSAIDs, cytostatic treatment, corticosteroids, nicotine inhalation
- Glossitis: Trimetoprim/sulfa
- Oral candidosis: Antibiotics, corticosteroid inhalation
- Gingival hyperplasia: Antiepileptics (phenytoin), immunosuppressant drugs, calcium channel antagonists (felodipin, amlodipin, nifedipin)

5.3.2 Treatment

There are different ways of treating dryness of the mouth. Drinking frequently and taking small sips can help but also chewing on ice cubes or small bits of fruit stimulates the production of saliva. Lubricant oral spray, chewing gum or oral gel, containing for example malic acid, can stimulate saliva secretion as long as there is still some saliva producing tissue left in the glands. This can help improve taste, enhance the appetite and facilitate speaking, chewing and swallowing.

When there is no saliva production left, replacement for saliva can be used to moisturise the dry membranes of the mouth and is often given in combination with sodium fluoride to protect the teeth.

It is also very important, if possible, to discontinue or lower the doses of drugs with anticholinergic effects; antihistamines, antipsychotics, antidepressants, urologic spasmolytics, anti-arrhythmics, drugs for Parkinson's disease and more. Prophylactic treatment against Candida infection, bacteria and caries can also be useful (Mouly et al. 2007).

It is vital to bear in mind that for the elderly mouth dryness has a negative impact on appetite, speech, oral hygiene, dental status and quality of life. It can be caused by many drugs used by old people and this must be considered when this problem occurs. Dry mouth should be prevented or treated in order to avoid permanent damages both to the membranes of the mouth and to the teeth.

5.4 Peptic Ulcers and Chronic Gastritis

Gastric ulcers, chronic gastritis and hiatus hernia are increasingly common conditions in old age. Both morbidity and mortality from bleeding stomach ulcers have increased in persons over 75 and this is in contrast to the lowered incidence in other age groups. It has been shown that the incidence of bleeding from ulcers increase significantly in individuals over 65 years and even more so in those aged 75 years or more (Zullo et al. 2007).

Aging is one of the major risk factors for developing gastric ulcers because of an increased incidence of Helicobacter pylori infections and a widely spread use of non-steroidal anti-inflammatory drugs (NSAID). Co-morbidity, with the need for prophylactic medication with antiplatelet therapy, warfarin and other anticoagulants, also increases the risk of gastrointestinal bleeding and ulcerations (Murakami et al. 1968).

Infection with Helicobacter pylori is widely spread in the world and as many as 50% of the population is estimated to be infected, with the highest incidence in Asia and developing countries. The bacterial toxins of Helicobacter pylori damage the epithelial cells in the stomach and can in the long term lead to gastric atrophy (Pilotto 1996, Faisal et al. 1990, Pilotto et al. 1999). The consequential decrease in secretion of acid causes a higher gastric pH level which can increase the risk of enteric infections, for example, with Campylobacter and Clostridium difficile.

Other risk factors for gastrointestinal bleedings are corticosteroids, anticoagulants and alcohol consumption. Tobacco and caffeine can both delay the healing of gastritis and ulcers (Box 5.2). Also many chronic diseases in old age need treatment with corticosteroids, e.g. for obstructive pulmonary disease, polymyalgia rheumatica or colitis. Corticosteroids themselves can cause gastrointestinal damage with bleeding and if they are used in combination with salicylic acid even in low doses the risk increases 4–6 folds. The widely spread use of prophylactic treatment with low doses of salicylic acid for many cardiovascular conditions adds to the risk of developing gastritis and gastric ulcers or bleeding from the intestines. The abdominal complications of NSAIDs include abdominal pain, gastritis, ulcers, bleeding, anemia and poor nutrition, as well as reduced quality of life (Hernández-Diaz and García-Rodriguez 2000).

Box 5.2 Drugs that increases the risk for gastritis, ulcers and esophagitis

Corticosteroids
Non-steroidal anti-inflammatory drugs
Salicylic acid
Anti-coagulants
Potassium salts
Alcohol
Tobacco
Caffeine
Nicotine

Non-steroidal anti-inflammatory drugs are frequently used by older persons for pain relief due to the high prevalence of degenerative and inflammatory joint diseases. The most common of these are osteoarthritis followed by rheumatoid arthritis, polymyalgia and gout. At ages over 70 years, osteoarthritis is common and almost half of the population has symptoms with stiffness and pain in joints and muscles that cause impaired functions. Non-steroidal anti-inflammatory drugs are effective for treating joint stiffness, swelling and pain caused by the arthritis but can be dangerous and even lethal. They are easily bought over the counter and are sold under many different names which can lead to double or triple medication within the same drug class.

The extensive use of NSAIDs in the older population can lead to serious and fatal health problems. See Box 5.3 for a case report on this problem. Damage to the stomach and intestines can occur without causing alarming symptoms and thus strike without warning. A serious side effect such as bleeding ulcers occurs more frequently when a combination with salicylic acid is given and even when used in low doses. Even though the risk of bleeding from the use of NSAIDs can be diminished by concomitant use of acid lowering drugs, such as proton pump inhibitors (PPI), antacids or H_2-receptor antagonists, the risk is still there.

Box 5.3 Case report on side effects of NSAIDs

A friend of mine is concerned about his 78 years old mother who has recently been to her doctor for an annual health check up. He is worried because at his mothers last visit her blood pressure had risen to 160/90 and she was prescribed an antihypertensive, a diuretic (thiazide). The medication is giving her a lot of problems due to the diuretic effect, and because of arthritis of the knees she moves slowly and this make it difficult for her to reach the bathroom in time. She has now developed urinary incontinence due to her medication.

Behind this lies a five year long history of arthritis of the knees with pain and stiffness and her problem has increased lately. She is in a lot of pain most of the time and the better periods are becoming shorter. She now has to use a cane when walking indoors and a perambulator when spending some time outdoors in her garden. She is unwilling to talk about this problem with her doctor because he has recommended her to have her knees operated on. So she has discussed her problem with her granddaughter who wants to help her.

The pharmacy provides a wide selection of different analgesics (pain killers) and her granddaughter chose a drug with anti inflammatory effects. This medication is a great help in relieving both her pain and joint stiffness due to arthritis. The drug should be taken one pill at a time three times daily but the old lady finds that if she takes 2 pills three times daily instead of 1 she can walk better and with less pain.

Problems:

- Her physician does not know about the medication with NSAIDs
- She has not personally been informed by the pharmacist of the side effects of the drug
- She is taking a too high dose of the drug and is unaware of the risks
- She is taking the NSAID drug for a longer time than recommended in old age (7–10 days at a time)
- She has developed hypertension from the NSAID medication
- The diuretic medication is giving her problem with incontinence that limits her social life
- The interaction between NSAID and diuretics is not taken into consideration

What to do?

Since she is in considerable pain the best alternative for this otherwise physically intact woman is an operation of her knees. In the meantime a supportive knee bandage can help relieve her pain in some way. She must tell her doctor that she is taking NSAIDs and be properly informed of the side effects and how to use the drug. The drug should only be used for short periods and in low doses because of the considerable danger of different side effects.

Adverse effects, which include gastritis, peptic ulcer, hypertension, kidney failure, delirium, bleeding diathesis and oedema of the lower extremities, are not uncommon. Most cases of knee arthritis can improve with the right kind of exercise of the thigh muscles, better personally adjusted walking aids and shoe implants can also be of help.

5.4.1 Treatment

The most widely used drug for this condition is proton pump inhibitors, PPI. Increasing amounts of PPIs are prescribed and also in some countries sold over the counter. Prescribing of different drugs within this class is in most countries among the ten most sold when measured both by number of prescriptions and DDDs (defined daily doses). The older population is often using PPIs for long term treatment and not according to the regime that is currently recommended, intermittent treatment for optimal symptom control. There are almost no severe side effects with PPIs but about 10% of the patients can experience constipation, diarrhoea, headache or flatulence. It is also important to know that a few cases of nephritis, disturbances in electrolytes (hyponatraemia, hypokalemia or hypomagnesaemia) and pancreatitis have been reported. Long term treatment can cause problems with malabsorption of, among other, calcium and vitamin B12 but so far this has not been sufficiently proved (Laine et al. 2000). Recently a study by Yang et al. 2006, has shown an increased incident of hip fractures among patients treated with PPIs. Other studies point at the risk of increased incidence of Clostridum difficile infections as well as community acquired pneumonia (Gulmez et al. 2007).

5.5 Hiatus Hernia

More and more people are inflicted by the condition of hiatus hernia, even more so in old age. The risk of experiencing symptoms of reflux esophagitis from hiatus hernia increases in old age and approximately half the population over 60 years of age can have a hiatus hernia to some degree (Manes et al. 2003). This condition is caused by a protrusion of the upper part of the stomach through the opening of the diaphragm and the hernia can occupy a large part of the chest cavity. Chronic heartburn, sour taste in the mouth when bending over or lying down and chest pain can be caused by this common condition. Besides the uncomfortable condition of esophagitis the symptoms can be confused with those of heart attacks or angina and lead to unnecessary examinations and drug treatment. Old people do not have the same clear symptoms as younger individuals and their risk for developing severe complications from hiatus hernia and esophagitis is higher (Kemppainen et al. 1997, Johnson and Fennerty 2004).

Furthermore, hiatus hernia with reflux esophagitis can cause scarring of the lower esophagus leading to difficulties in swallowing, increased risk of cancer and anaemia caused by slow chronic bleeding from the inflammatory tissue. In very old and sick people the risk of hiatus hernia causing pneumonia due to aspiration of stomach secretions into the lungs, increases. This can easily happen when they lie down without elevation of the upper part of the body. Besides old age, other common risk factors for developing hiatus hernia are obesity, pulmonary diseases with frequent hard coughing, constipation, heavy lifting, vomiting, heredity and smoking.

5.5.1 Treatment

Avoiding drugs and other contributors that increase the acid secretion and reflux can be combined with changes in the intake of foods and stimulants (Box 5.4). Surgery is needed in the more severe cases but is very seldom used. Treatment with acid lowering drugs, such as proton pump inhibitors (PPI), antacids or H_2-receptor antagonists, can relieve the symptoms of reflux esophagitis but not treat the cause, hiatus hernia. Sleeping with the upper part of the body slightly elevated, about 20–25 cm (8–10 inches), can decrease the symptoms and diminish the risk of aspiration to the lungs.

Box 5.4 What to avoid for not worsening the reflux condition

Drugs:

- NSAIDs
- Intestinal antispasmodics
- Calcium channel blockers
- Antidepressants

Intake of:

- Nicotine
- Caffeine
- Alcohol
- Fatty foods
- Large meals

Others:

- Frequently bending over
- Heavy lifting
- Constipation with the need of straining
- Obesity
- Sleeping without elevation of the head

Finally be aware of the fact that diseases in the upper part of the gastrointestinal tract are common in the elderly and can cause severe complications and even be fatal. Drugs that are often used in the elderly due to chronic diseases with inflammation and pain are often the cause of gastritis, peptic ulcers and hiatus hernia. The risks of medication side effects as a reason for the problem must be taken into account when treating elderly for peptic ulcers and stomach pain.

5.6 Urinary Incontinence

Among elderly women as much as 80% suffer from involuntary voiding of the bladder, urinary incontinence (UI). In the United States approximately 12.5 million people are affected by incontinence and a European study showed a prevalence of between 12% and 22% in all ages and an increase to 30–40% in ages over 75 years (Hampel et al. 1997). Women experience UI twice as often as men. Incontinence becomes more common in old age, with existing co-morbidity of all kinds and life styles (Box 5.5). There are different forms of urinary incontinence and they differ in cause and treatment. This problem causes not only personal distress but also a considerable cost for society as a whole (Jackson 1997). Lower quality of life is often reported in people with UI and the risk increases by the withdrawal from social interaction and participation in sports and other activities. An estimated cost for the care of patients with UI in the United States was approximately 26 billion dollars in year 1995 (Wagner and Hu 1998). Other studies have come up with a calculated cost that represents two percent of the total national health budget.

Box 5.5 Risk factors for urinary incontinence

Age
Child births
Number of pregnancies
Hysterectomy
Obesity
Smoking
Hormone changes, menopause
Diuretics
Non-steroid inflammatory drugs
Corticosteroids

Of all people with UI, half of them have stress incontinence, about one fifth urge incontinence and one third a mix of the two conditions. With more advanced age incontinence due to central and/or peripheral nervous damages tends to increase. Other circumstances such as mobility disorders, impaired eye sight and balance disturbances also make it harder for elderly women to reach the bathroom in time and leakage occurs (Payne 1998).

5.6.1 Stress Urinary Incontinence

Physical strain that increases the abdominal pressure such as coughing, sneezing, jumping or even laughing can cause urinary leakage due to the lack of closing capacity of the muscles surrounding the urethra. The capacity to close the peripheral urethra completely is vital to avoid stress UI. The incapacity to close the sphincter is due to changes in the hormonal production in women during menopause leading to weakening of the connective tissue and muscles surrounding the urethra. The incontinence due to this weakening is treated with regular exercise of the pelvic floor muscles. It takes intensive, regular and instructed exercises for a long period of time to reach positive longstanding results, otherwise relapses are common. Another form of treatment that often is successful for overweight people is losing weight. A surgical procedure of the pelvic floor is a simple treatment but surgery is often more successful in younger women. Younger women are often helped by surgery, around 80%, but as the women get older (over 75 years) the results are less promising.

5.6.2 Overactive Bladder/Urge Incontinence

An overactive bladder gives the patient an urgent need to urinate and often leads to leakage. Urinary muscle spasms give the urge to urinate even though the amount of urine is comparatively small. With age, the capacity of the bladder to contain or hold the urine becomes lesser and it signals for micturation at much smaller quantities. Both day and night this leads to shorter time periods between voiding of the bladder.

Oedema of the lower extremities often accumulates during the day time and the superfluous tissue fluids are absorbed during the night due to the horizontal position of the body and the rise in filtration capacity in the kidneys. This form of nightly voiding of the bladder can be alleviated by using compression stockings that prevent daytime swelling in the legs.

5.6.2.1 Treatment

Most of the treatment options mentioned in Box 5.6 are often needed to be used and in combination to help solve the problem. The effect of anticholinergic drugs on urge incontinence is often small and disappointing. If no positive effects are seen in a two weeks trial period of treatment the drugs are not likely to help at all and the medication should be discontinued. Side effects are common with these drugs and besides the peripheral anticholinergic effects, the negative effects on the central nervous system should also be considered. The frequently occurring peripheral anticholinergic effects are dryness of the mouth, constipation, blurred vision and tremors. Very few studies on the treatment of urge incontinence have confirmed what side effects these spasmolytic anticholinergic drugs have on the brain in older people. Other studies have shown negative effects of anticholinergic drugs on the cognitive functions (even confusional states can be triggered) in individuals over 65 years of age, especially when used in combination with other anticholinergic medications (Chapple 2000, Andersson 1997).

Box 5.6 Treatment options for urinary incontinence

Exercises to strengthen the pelvic floor muscles
Behavioural therapy
Anticholinergic drugs
Desmopressin
Modified drinking habits (lower intake of fluids in the evening, avoiding certain fluids)
Operation

Both food and drinks can worsen the symptoms of UI by diverse mechanisms; overfilling of the bladder, irritation of the mucosal membrane of the bladder, promote infections, stimulating the production of urine or interfering with the brain's signals to the bladder (Box 5.7).

Box 5.7 Examples of mechanisms that can cause urinary incontinence

Overfilling of the bladder:

- too high intake of fluids; if more than 2 litres (2.11 quarts) of fluids a day is consumed the risk increase of imbalance between intake and urine production
- incapacity to empty the bladder caused be e.g. hypertrophy of the prostate

Irritating the mucosal membrane of the bladder:

- too little fluid makes the urine concentrated and also increases the risk for infections
- acidic foods and drinks, e.g. coffee, tea, tomatoes, citrus fruits, sugared drinks, carbonated drinks, spicy food

Stimulating the production of urine:

- caffeine containing drinks; coffee, tea, colas, chocolate
- alcoholic beverages; interferes with the brain's signal to the bladder

5.6.3 Drugs and Urinary Incontinence

How can medications make incontinence symptoms worse? A number of different drug classes can have side effects that worsen the symptoms of incontinence and are the major reason for incontinence in the patients. There are several different ways for how drugs can increase symptoms of incontinence. Some examples are mentioned here.

- increased urine output (diuretics, caffeine)
- increased oedema (calcium channel blockers, NSAID, corticosteroids)
- relaxation of the bladder (cholinesterase inhibitors)
- reduced awareness of the need to urinate (sedatives, alcohol)
- reduced capacity for emptying of the bladder (antidepressants, anticholinergic drugs)

The side effects of drugs can lead to restricted ability of the bladder to contract, relaxing the bladder muscles or decrease the patient's awareness of the need to urinate. Retention of urine in the bladder is a very common side effect for some drugs and this increases the risks for infections and kidney failure (Box 5.8). It is always important for the health care professional to be aware of medication as a risk factor and to reassess their usefulness when the patient is suffering from urinary incontinence. The best alternative is to stop the medications involved and if this is not possible a change to other drugs without these side effects should be considered. In some cases the symptoms can be relieved by lowering the doses of the compromising drugs.

Box 5.8 Drugs that can increase or cause urinary incontinence

Diuretics
Calcium channel blockers
Non-steroid inflammatory drugs
Corticosteroids
Sedatives
Cholinesterase inhibitors
Antidepressants
Vitamin C

5.7 Renal Failure in Old Age

Both females and males experience age-related problems from the urinary tracts, for example prostate hypertrophy in men and urinary incontinence in women. Kidney problems become more frequent in old age not only because of the normal functional decline but as a result of diseases associated with aging, and their treatment.

The normal way of excreting toxic metabolites and excess fluids in the body is through the kidneys but these also produce vital substances that can control different functions in the body such as vitamin D, renin and erythropoietin. Besides the normal decline in renal function with old age, a number of chronic diseases common in the elderly also affect the function of the kidneys in a negative way. Examples of common chronic diseases in old age that can cause kidney dysfunction are hypertension, diabetes and gout. Old people are more prone to experience symptoms of dehydration when feverish, famished or injured and this is caused by their lesser capacity to concentrate the urine. Drugs that cause loss of blood circulation to the kidneys can all induce renal failure, especially in emergency situations with high risk of dehydration and/or hypotension. An important consequence of the impaired renal function that occurs in old age is the disability to excrete drugs which increases the risk of drug-accumulation and adverse drug reactions (see also Chapter 2).

There are also drugs which by themselves can cause kidney failure. The mechanisms behind drugs negative effects on the kidneys are multiple. Among the most important is diminished blood flow to the kidneys (prerenal failure). Others are immunological damages to the nephrons caused by deposition of autoimmune complexes or direct nephrotoxicity caused by for example, antibiotics. The kidney function can also be damaged by post-renal obstructions, for example, kidney stones, urethral strictures or prostate hyperplasia (Ashley 2004).

Examples of how medication can cause renal failure:

- Diuretics; especially loop diuretics, can cause blood volume depletion
- NSAIDs; lowers the blood flow through the kidneys (worsen pre-renal failure)
- ACE inhibitors; altered renal hemodynamic regulation (renal failure)
- Combinations of ACE-inhibitors, diuretics and NSAIDs highly increase the risk
- Excessive use of laxatives can result in renal failure

5.7.1 Drugs that Can Increase the Risk of Renal Failure

5.7.1.1 ACE-Inhibitors

Angiotensin converting enzymes- inhibitors (ACE-inhibitors) are a group of drugs that are very potent in dilating the blood vessels and through this mechanism lower the blood pressure. Therefore they can also improve heart function in patients with heart failure. In some cases they are also used for preventing renal failure in persons with hypertension and/or diabetes. Paradoxically, this later use of ACE-inhibitors has caused an increasing amount of cases of acute renal failure, especially in older patients and patients with other risk factors for renal failure. With combinations of ACE-inhibitors and NSAIDs there can in a very short period of treatment be irreversible kidney damage. In emergency situations where drop in blood pressure or dehydration often occurs there is a high risk of renal shutdown with serious consequences for the patients.

The use of ACE-inhibitors can also lead to an increased risk of developing high levels of potassium and often do so when given in combination with aldosterone, amiloride or potassium salts and this increase the risk for arrhythmias. Besides ACE-inhibitors the angiotensin II antagonist drugs can have the same negative impact on renal hemodynamic regulation.

5.7.1.2 NSAIDs

A common cause of renal failure in the elderly is the use of NSAIDs and it occurs more frequently in women. One to five percent of treatment with NSAIDs leads to some kind of renal dysfunction and mostly vasomotor acute renal failure occurs (Bakris and Kern 1989, Griffin et al. 2000, Henry et al. 1997).

These drugs are the most prescribed medicines in the world. For certain NSAIDs, ibuprofen and indomethacin, there has been shown a dose response relation for renal failure risk. For individual NSAIDs, those with longer half lives than 12 hours have proved to be more dangerous. There has not been shown any clear advantages for selective cox-2-inhibition to the more unselective in this aspect.

5.7.1.3 How to Prevent Progressive Renal Failure Due to Medication

To be able to decide when to adjust current medication use in elderly patients with rising creatinine levels it can be helpful to estimate GFR (glomerular filtration rate) by using the Cockcroft and Gault equation, see Chapter 2. It is vital to respond quickly when the creatinine level has risen above 30–50% of the baseline value from when, for example, starting the patient on ACE-inhibitors, digoxin or metformin. For drugs with mainly renal elimination it is in most situations to the benefit for the patients to adjust drug doses and in some cases change to medications with less negative renal effects (Matzke and Frye 1997). It is easier to decide what measures to take concerning medication when the patient is in a stable phase of a chronic disease and the creatinine level is raised but not progressing. But the risk for severe renal failure in emergency situations must be considered and steps be taken to immediately assess the risk for renal damage due to drugs such as digoxin, metformin, ACE-inhibitors, antibiotics, diuretics, phenytoin and NSAIDs. It is also essential to avoid dehydration and low blood pressure which can cause fatal renal failure.

Finally be aware of the fact that more and more drugs are used by the elderly that can have negative effects on the kidney function. Anti-hypertensive drugs are often needed to reach lower blood pressure levels in the elderly but this can increase the risk of severe renal failure. The risk of renal dysfunction caused by drugs increases with the normal decline in glomerular filtration rate that occurs in old age.

5.8 Obstruction of Urinary Flow

Drug therapy with various drugs can cause lowered urine flow through the kidneys with at times irreparable damages. Anticoagulants can cause bleedings and resulting blood clots can obstruct the urine filtration on different levels in the kidneys. Retroperitoneal fibrosis can be caused by several drug classes such as betablockers, methyldopa, ergot derivates and bromocriptine and can lead to obstructions in the urine flow.

Other drugs can cause hypercalcaemia and increase the risk of forming kidney stones that can damage the kidneys and ureters and cause infections. Examples are cytostatic agents, sulphonamides, radiological contrast media, statins (through rhabdomyolysis), vitamin D and intake of calcium and antacids.

5.9 Falls and Fractures

Injuries related to falls are an often re-occurring health problem in elderly people. Almost one third of persons over 65 years of age fall at least once a year and half of these are more frequent fallers. About ten percent of the casualties in emergency wards are due to damages caused by falling and most of them are elderly persons over 65. This results in a very high economic burden for the health care systems all over the world. Among the most serious injuries caused by falling are haemorrhages in the brain and hip fractures. Dizziness, impaired balance and poor eye sight, as well as a multitude of chronic diseases, can increase the risk of damages from falls. Besides the sometimes grave somatic injuries related to falls, falling also has an impact on the quality of life, social interaction and mental health in general (Koski et al.1996).

The majority of fractures in the aging populations are caused by low impact violence such as a fall caused by slipping indoors. Many falls happen when getting out of bed, walking indoors or falling to the floor from a chair. The surroundings are often indoors and it happens in their own apartment or house. Both somatic and environmental causes of falls and following fractures must be examined and their possible association with current pharmacotherapy.

What associations can there be between falls in old age and drugs? During the last decades, a number of scientific studies have been performed to examine if there are associations or not (Blalock et al. 2005, Leipzig et al. 1999a,b). Several of these studies have shown that many different kinds of drugs increase the numbers of falls and especially in people 65 years or older. These falls can lead to both physical injuries and mental health problems in elderly with consequences for a long time afterwards.

There are many different reasons why elderly people fall more easily than young people do. Chronic diseases often give rise to general weakness, less muscle strength and impaired balance which all can make falling more dangerous (Box 5.9).

Box 5.9 Risk factors for falls

Joint disease (osteoarthritis, rheumatoid arthritis, gout)
Depression
Orthostatic hypotension
Cognitive dysfunction
Impaired eye sight
Impaired balance and walking abilities
Muscle weakness
Use of fall-risk increasing drugs
Use of polypharmacy ($\geq$ 5 drugs)

Drugs also play a prominent role as a risk factor for causing falls due to vertigo, hypotension, orthostatic reactions, sedation, blurred eye sight, muscle weakness and other common side effects. There are both specific drug classes and polypharmacy causing side effects that can lead to higher risk of falling in the patients (Box 5.10).

Box 5.10 Examples of drug classes that can increase the number of falls

Antidepressants
Antipsychotics
Sedatives (benzodiazepines)
Tranquilizers
Diuretics
Antiepileptic

Mainly drugs used for cardiovascular diseases and psychotropic medication have falls as a side effect but also other drug classes are involved. The side effects that are most dangerous are those that lead to sedation, vertigo, orthostatic reactions or hypotension, impaired balance or poor eye sight and cognitive reduction. The side effects can be caused either by the drug itself or by interactions between drugs, or between drugs and illness, and by polypharmacy. If a fall leads to injuries or not is due to a number of circumstances of which the most important ones are mentioned in Box 5.11.

Box 5.11 Factors that increase the risk of injuries from falling

The amount of energy involved when falling and the height of the fall
Falling against hard obstacles
Falling backwards or sideways
Mass, quality, size and strength of the bones in the body
Absorption by the body of the impact, this varies due to the amount of soft tissue between the blow and the bones
Balance and neuromuscular reflexes to protect against the fall
The presence of dizziness, sedatives, alcohol, acute and chronic diseases

5.9.1 Fall Prevention

Fall preventive interventions that have been tested and shown to reduce the incidence of falls are mentioned in Box 5.12 (Tinetti 2003, Gillespie et al. 2009, Howe et al. 2007). It is important to make an individual assessment for each person and to draw up an individual plan to reduce hers/his risk factors. A multifactor approach has shown the most benefits for patients and when successful, it can reduce the number of falls by 35–40%. A lot can be gained by taking regular physical exercises such as muscle and balance strengthening by walking, dancing or swimming. Physical training in groups is overall often more effective than individual training programmes but this must be assessed for each person separately. The knowledge of effective interventions has to be more widespread in health care institutions and when an elderly person falls it is important to understand the warning sign, especially, as there are now methods to be taken and recommended to prevent future accidents and damages (Box 5.12).

Box 5.12 Interventions tested and to some extent shown to reduce the incidence of falls

Multidisciplinary and multifactor intervention programmes
Systematic medication revision (lower dosages, withdrawals or change of drugs)
Exercises for muscle strengthening and balance training (e.g. Tai Chi, group exercise, brisk walking, dancing)
Home hazard assessment and modification
Withdrawal of psychotropic medication
Nutritional supplements
Vitamin D supplements
Individual information and education on exercises and reducing fall risks
Correction of visual deficiency

Finally hold in mind that falls are frequent in old age and can lead to severe consequences, including sufferings both for the individual and the next of kin. Also the cost for the society of falls and fractures are considerable. Falls increase with the use of fall-risk-increasing drugs and polypharmacy and can be prevented by a multifactor approach including reassessing the medications used by older people.

5.10 Osteoporosis

Osteoporosis is a world wide problem with consequences for both the individual affected and society as a whole. Osteoporosis affects an estimated 75 million people in Europe, USA and Japan. The estimated cost for the treatment of osteoporosis in the world is 18.3 billion dollars a year. Hip, vertebrae and wrist are the most frequent sites for osteoporotic fractures. Due to the increase in the population over 60 years of age this scenario is about to escalate and regarding one of the most serious fractures, the hip fracture, an increase with more than 200% is likely to occur. Today, approximately 1.6 million hip fractures happen yearly in the world and, in the nearest forty to fifty years, this number can increase to about 5 million. The risk of hip fractures is highest in Norway, Iceland, Sweden, Denmark and the United States (NIH 2000).

Osteoporosis is in many ways a silent disease and osteoporotic fractures occurs mainly in women, the ratio being 1.6 females to 1 male. There are many risk factors that have been identified as increasing the development of osteoporosis and age, sex and life styles factors are some (Box 5.13)

Box 5.13 Risk factors for developing osteoporosis

Age
Sex
Heredity
Ethnicity
Low physical activity
Earlier low impact fractures
Medication
Drugs
Smoking
Alcohol
Early menopause
Body length

There are no symptoms of the poor bone quality until a fracture occurs. When a person has reached the age of 80 the bone quality has in most cases deteriorated to the extent to put her/him at high risk of developing a fracture. Osteoporosis occurs when there is an imbalance between resorption and rebuilding of the bone. In youth, the maximum bone mass index is reached and the amount of physical activity before 20 years of age is of great importance for bone quality in later life.

The definition of osteoporosis is (NIH 2000): "A systemic skeletal disease characterized by low bone mass and micro architectural deterioration of bone tissue, with a consequent increase in bone fragility and susceptibility to fracture".

Also definitions on different stages of reduced bone quality has been made by the WHO study group; diagnostic categories for different stages of the disease.

- Osteopenia (low bone mass): BMD between 1 and 2.5 SD below young adult mean
- Osteoporosis: BMD 2.5 SD or more below the young adult mean
- Severe osteoporosis: BMD 2.5 SD or more below the young adult mean and one or more fragility fractures

The human bone can be measured with dual X-ray absorptometry (DXA scanning) and a score for bone mass/mineral density (BMD) is then achieved and compared to peak bone mass in young individuals with a normal bone structure. A study group for WHO (World Health Organisation) has developed a tool, FRAX® (WHO 1994), for evaluating the risk of fractures in patients with osteoporosis. It integrates the risks associated with clinical factors with those of the measured BMD at the femoral neck. This tool can be helpful when making decisions on treatment and calculating the prognosis for individual patients (WHO 1994, Kanis et al. 2002).

Primary osteoporosis is the most common form of the condition. The secondary form of osteoporosis is diagnosed when an illness and/or medications are present with a negative impact on BMD. Examples of common chronic conditions in old people that can cause secondary osteoporosis are seen in Box 5.14. Examples of drugs that can cause secondary osteoporosis are glucocorticoids, too high doses of thyroid hormone, anticonvulsants, and heparin. Especially the use of glucocorticoids has been known to cause severe osteoporosis even within a short period of treatment. Depending on the doses the development of osteoporosis can occur within a few weeks or months.

Box 5.14 Examples of conditions that can cause secondary osteoporosis

Hyperthyroidism
Hyperparathyroidism
Hypogonadism
Cushing's syndrome
Alcohol abuse
Diabetes
Rheumatoid arthritis
Multiple myeloma

Malnutrition can also cause secondary osteoporosis in persons with different deficiencies of substances such as calcium and vitamin D. Malnutrition due to starvation caused by most severe or terminal chronic diseases and malabsorption due to inflammatory bowel diseases (colitis, Mb Crohn) can give rise to rapidly diminishing bone tissue.

5.10.1 Symptoms and Signs of Osteoporosis

Even though this silent progressive disease in its early stages does not give rise to any symptoms, the signs can be seen later on. Weight bearing parts of the spine and hips are especially prone to fractures and deformation. The body length of an osteoporotic woman decreases significantly because of bone loss in the vertebrae. Also, a deformation of the spine occurs which can cause problems such as muscle weakness, balance disturbances, walking difficulties and even breathing problems. Smaller movements as sneezing, bending or rising from a chair can be enough to cause a fracture. When a fracture occurs pain is a usual sign and often becomes chronic. The most common location for osteoporotic pain is mainly in the back and the ribs. Pain in combination with fear of recurrent falling and fractures can in the worst cases lead to mental illness, depression, social isolation and anxiety (Cooper et al. 1993, Cummings and Melton 2002).

5.10.2 Treatment

Treatment should focus on primary preventive actions taken against developing clinically evident osteoporosis. When a fracture has already occurred, and this is often when the diagnosis of osteoporosis is finally reached, secondary prevention should be considered. Adequate intake or supplementation with calcium and vitamin D in combination with physical activity and exposure to sunshine, are the basis for all treatments for osteoporosis. Depending on age, bone density and number of risk factors, further actions should be considered. Among these are medication with alendronate, risedronate, etidronate, strontium ranelat, raloxifen or teriparatide and the most favourable treatment must be individually chosen. A problem with the usage of these drugs for osteoporosis, and calcium and vitamin D supplements, is the side effects that often lead to low compliance.

Note that osteoporosis is a worldwide problem that increases due to the aging of all populations. It is important to diagnose osteoporosis early in order to prevent its progression and lessen the economic consequences for the society. Osteoporosis can be caused or worsened by medications and this should be avoided. Pain from fractures and deformation of the spine often has grave consequences for the individual and can be avoided by a combination of lifestyle changes and appropriate medical treatment.

5.11 Sarcopenia, Muscle Weakness in Old Age

As we grow older our muscle strength diminishes and the risk of developing sarcopenia increases. The meaning of the word sarcopenia is an abnormal decline in muscle strength and mass. Another word is muscle atrophy. Between early middle age and older age the mean decrease is 50% of muscle mass. Another way to calculate the loss of muscle mass is that over 50 years of age 1–2% of muscle tissue mass vanishes yearly. Between 50 and 70 years of age almost 15% of muscle strength per 10 years disappears. The resulting disability in older persons with sarcopenia has been calculated to cost approximately 900 dollars per person and year. The yearly total of healthcare expenditures for sarcopenia in the United States is estimated at 18–20 billions (Janssen et al. 2004).

The concept of sarcopenia is not as well known as osteoporosis, which is the equivalent in bone tissue loss. Even though an older patient has not lost weight, sarcopenia can still be present because of an increased amount of fat tissue. It is important to check the patients for muscle strength as this is a condition which we are able to treat successfully if discovered in time. There are several other reasons for loss of muscle strength in the elderly, such as sickness, inactivity and poor nutrition (Doherty 2003).

The normal loss of muscle strength in the process of aging is caused by a combination of factors, both genetically and life style components. The life style factors are physical inactivity and low intake of nutritional agents of which protein is the most important.

The production of both anabolic sex hormones and growth hormone decreases in aging and the result is muscle loss. Also the loss of neural motor cells gives rise to atrophy of the muscles. In the aging process an increased inflammatory activity can be seen and it causes degeneration of muscle tissue through insuline resistance and activation of protein breakdown enzymes. The increased inflammatory activity is due to both normal aging as well as the presence of multiple chronic diseases (Dutta 1997.

Drugs that increase sedation and give muscle relaxation can have a negative effect on muscle strength and the ability to maintain physical activity, for example, benzodiazepines and other tranquilizers. Corticosteroids have a well known side effect on muscle tissue that leads to muscle atrophy and increases with the dosage.

There is no other way to diminish the effects of sarcopenia but to maintain and increase physical activities and it is vital to keep a good nutritional strategy, especially in old age (Binder et al. 2005, Ades et al. 1996, Evans 1995). The way to be successful in this is to take up these habits early in life and be aware of the risks of inactivity.

5.12 Orthostatic Hypotension

The most studied component of blood pressure disturbances in the elderly is by far, high blood pressure. Only a very few scientific experiments have been performed on low blood pressure in the elderly. This is, among other reasons, due to the differences in severity and long term prognosis of the two conditions. Research on high blood pressure has high priority also because of the financial interest from the drug companies to develop new drugs in this field. Hypotension, low blood pressure, can be both a disturbing health problem and dangerous to the individual. It can be dangerous because of the increased risk of damages from fainting and falling.

Orthostatic reactions is defined as a symptomatic fall in blood pressure and it is measured by a fall in systolic blood pressure by ≥20 mmHg or to below 90 after three minutes of standing up after lying down (The Consensus Committee 1996). Orthostatic hypotension is estimated to prevail in 18–28% of the population over 65 and in public health surveys as many as 25% of persons over 80 years experienced symptoms related to low blood pressure and orthostatic reactions (Colledge et al. 1994, Brignole 1998).

In people with orthostatic hypotension there is a dysfunction in the capacity to adapt to changes in blood pressure when the body changes positions (Verhaeverbeke and Mets 1997). Changes in the autonomic nerve system give rise to an incapacity to react with a baroreflex mediated vasoconstriction and increase the heart rate which is the normal reaction to changes in body position from lying or sitting to standing upright. Besides these changes in old age of compensating reactions, medications have a substantial role in causing orthostatic hypotension. An increased prevalence of neurodegenerative diseases, for example, Parkinson's disease and dementia, also gives rise to autonomic dysfunction.

The symptoms of orthostatic reactions can lead to lower quality of life caused by anxiety for injuries from fainting and/or falling. Other symptoms are; syncope (8%), feeling of weakness (22%), dizziness (22%) and disturbances in vision and hearing (19%), palpitations and sweating (30%), pain in neck, shoulders and chest (10%). The deprivation of oxygen and blood to the heart and brain worsens the condition and in severe cases can cause irreparable damages (Montastruc et al. 1997, Pavri and Ho 2003).

Different causes are seen for this condition, including: low blood volume (due to, for example, dehydration, overuse of diuretics, anaemia or bleeding), relocation of the blood volume (varicose veins, postprandial symptoms), heart failure, long term immobilisation or drugs (diuretics, antihypertensives, antipsychotics).

Many different drug classes have shown to cause hypotension and orthostatic reactions and drugs for cardiovascular conditions, psychoactive medicines and polypharmacy, can all have this side effect (Box 5.15). Among the most frequently used drugs in the elderly are diuretics, ACE-inhibitors, angiotensin II antagonists, calcium channel blockers and antidepressants.

Box 5.15 Drugs that can increase the risk of hypotension

Diuretics
Antihypertensive drugs
Heart medication, betablockers, ACE-inhibitors, long acting nitro derivates, calcium channel blockers, angiotensin II antagonists

Antipsychotics
Drugs for Parkinson's disease
Tricyclic and SSRI antidepressants
Drugs for erectile dysfunction
Narcotics
Alcohol

Many chronic diseases can cause hypotension. Heart conditions (and drugs used for its treatment) can lead to bradycardia, thyroid dysfunction (either under- or over activity), diabetes mellitus, Parkinson's disease and neuropathies. Also, all acute conditions with the risk of dehydration, such as fever, vomiting, diarrhoea and bleeding, can cause hypotension.

5.12.1 Treatment

For elderly patients it is important to take precautions to compensate for orthostatic hypotension because of the higher risk of injuries from syncopation and falling. To receive individual advice on how to prevent this reaction is the best way to make the patient feel in control of the situation instead of being scared and passive. The simple advice of keeping two glasses of water by the bed and drinking them before getting up in the morning, or better still, be served breakfast with plenty of liquids in bed, can solve parts of the problem. It is also important to take some time (5–10 minutes) to adjust to the upright position by remaining sitting up on the bed before standing up and walking away. An increased intake of salt, for example by drinking bouillon instead of water, lesser intake of depleting drinks such as coffee or tea, can also help. The use of compression stockings has in practice been shown to alleviate the problem of hypotension but not enough scientific evidence is at hand at the moment. In severe cases these measures are not enough and drugs to make the blood pressure rise are necessary to prescribe (Oldenburg et al. 2002). For example, in cases with low blood pressure due to Parkinson's disease, the substance midodrine has been used. NSAIDs have side effects that lead to higher blood pressure and if the patients do not have any risk factors for the use of anti-inflammatory drugs, this can be tried. Fludrocortisone is normally used for treating Addison's disease but as hypertension is a common side effect it has been used for severe symptomatic orthostatic hypotension as well. Other side effects of fludrocortisone are oedema, heart enlargement and heart failure. There are many old patients that can not be treated with drugs against hypotension without considerable risks because they often suffer from heart conditions and renal failure (Mathias and Kimber 1998, Podoleanu et al. 2006). Hence it is important to be familiar with different ways of treating this condition in order to help the elderly patients without risking side effects. See Box 5.16 for available treatments options.

Box 5.16 Treatment options for hypotension

Reassessment of current pharmacotherapy
Salt, sodium intake
Water, increased water intake leads to higher blood volume and prevent dehydration
Compression stockings
Increased physical activity
Drugs: fludrocortisone, NSAIDs, midodrine, pyridostigmine, caffeine

It is important to be aware of the fact that orthostatic hypotension is a common condition in the elderly and can lead to injuries and lowered quality of life. Drug treatment for cardiovascular, neurological and psychiatric disorders can cause hypotension as a side effect. The treatment of orthostatic hypotension should be concentrated on behavioural adaptation, intake of water and salt and in some cases drug treatment is necessary.

5.13 Vertigo

A common ailment in old age is the unpleasant sensation of dizziness, faintness, imbalance or light-headedness and a general feeling of unsteadiness. It is the most common complaint from old people when consulting a physician. Almost 18% of the population over 65 years of age suffers from vertigo. It is more common in women and the prevalence increases with age. In the very old, over 85 years, as many as 50% complain about some form of vertigo and it is a risk factor for functional decline (Colledge et al. 1994). The causes of vertigo symptoms can roughly be split up into two different categories. The first category describes where the symptoms originate from; the peripheral or central vestibular system. The second category describes for how long the symptom prevails; continuous or episodic. This can be useful when deciding on how the examination of the patient shall be performed and what treatments there are available to help the patient (Davis 1994, Jonsson et al. 2004, Uneri and Polat 2008). The cause of vertigo can be due to both peripheral and central vestibular dysfunctions.

The most prevalent peripheral cause of this symptom is benign paroxysmal positional vertigo (BPPV) followed by ototoxity due to drugs or environmental substances. BPPV gives rise to short periods of often intense and very unpleasant feelings of dizziness, spinning and sometimes nausea. It starts when the position of the head is changed, for example when turning in bed or getting out of bed or bending the head. In elderly persons this is usually due to a shift of calcium crystals debris in the inner ear labyrinths, situated in the semicircular canals. This reason for BPPV is one of the few treatable causes of episodic vertigo.

In all patients and ages BPPV can also be an effect of damage to the peripheral vestibular system by a head trauma, ear infection or ototoxicity. Ototoxity can be a result of different drugs or chemicals in the surrounding environment.

Examples of drugs that can give permanent damage to the inner ear or acoustic nerve are antibiotics (aminoglycosides) and chemotherapy (cisplatin). Other more commonly used drugs can give reversible ototoxity with vertigo.

In most cases the side effects of drugs causing orthostatic hypotension is reversible but all the same unpleasant and dangerous to frail elderly patients. Commonly used drugs that can cause vertigo are antihypertensives (ACE-inhibitors, angiotensin II antagonists), diuretics, (frusemide), analgesics (acetyl salicylic acid, tramadol, opioids), antiepileptics (phenytoin, carbamazepine), and alcohol.

In the elderly other reasons for episodic vertigo can be transient ischemic attacks, heart arrhythmias or viral infections causing vestibular neuritis.

The most common causes of continuous central vertigo are medication, brain damages due to stroke or dementia, cerebellar atrophy and psychological reactions. It can also be a symptom of general cerebral ischemia due to hypotension, medication or cardiac arrhythmia.

5.13.1 Treatment

There are not many ways of helping elderly patients who suffer from vertigo and in cases with severe problems the condition is disabling and can cause functional decline and cognitive dysfunction. One exception from this is the most common cause for BPPV, the dislocation of the calcium crystals in the semicircular canals in the inner ear labyrinth, which can be treated with an exercise called the Epley manoeuvre. This can be taught to the patient by a physiotherapist and consists of a series of movements of the body and head, aiming to remove dislocated crystals and debris from the canal which then later are absorbed.

Both for peripheral and central causes of vertigo it is essential to reassess all current medications and to test for orthostatic hypotension. The risk of falls and injuries can be lowered by reducing doses, changing into more favourable drugs without side effects causing dizziness or hypotension and to avoid or reduce polypharmacy. For most patients with vertigo they are helped by correction of vision and hearing and also to be provided with walking aids. This enables the patients to be more active both indoors and outdoors. Physical exercise, including specific balance training, muscle strengthening and improving coordination, is advantageous in many ways for elderly, especially those suffering from dizziness. To make life safer and lessen the risk for falls home hazards should also be removed.

Medications for symptomatic relief from vertigo consist of antiemetics, benzodiazepines and antihistamines. They are all mostly aimed at the psychological consequences of dizziness and can all have highly unfavourable side effects, for example, sedation, anticholinergic effects and insomnia. The psychological consequences of dizziness in elderly should rather be treated with information about the condition, supportive help actions and increased social activities, than with drugs.

Vertigo is a disabling condition common in the elderly and a physical examination including blood pressure measurements is necessary to determine whether orthostatic hypotension is present or not. Commonly used drugs can be the cause of vertigo and reassessment of the medication should be made regularly. The condition can be diminished by exercises for balance, coordination and muscle strengthening. Psychological reactions to vertigo are common and must be dealt with to make the patients more secure and willing to lead an active life.

5.14 Conclusions

- Constipation is common in old age and have often negative effects on both health and quality of life
- Constipation is often caused by chronic diseases and by many different drugs and is best treated by life style changes
- Mouth dryness has a negative impact on appetite, speech, oral hygiene, dental status and quality of life
- Dry mouth can be caused by most drugs used by old people and should be prevented or treated to avoid permanent damages
- Diseases in the upper part of the gastrointestinal tract are common in the elderly and can cause severe complications and even be fatal
- The risks of medication side effects must be taken into account when treating elderly for peptic ulcers and stomach pain
- Urinary incontinence causes both distress for the individual and a substantial economic burden on the society
- Urinary incontinence can be caused and worsened by drug treatment for diverse chronic conditions and should be treated with a multifactor aim
- The risk of renal dysfunction caused by drugs increases with the normal decline in glomerular filtration rate that occurs in old age
- The increased risk of renal failure in the elderly must be considered when prescribing drugs that are dependent on the renal function for excretion
- Falls are frequent in old age and can lead to sufferings both for the individual and the next of kin. It also causes a high economic burden on society
- Falls increase with the use of fall-risk-increasing drugs and polypharmacy and can be prevented by improving the medications used by older people
- Osteoporosis is a worldwide problem that increases due to the aging of all populations
- Osteoporosis can be caused or worsened by medications
- Fractures and deformations can be avoided by a combination of lifestyle changes and appropriate medical treatment
- The normal course in aging is loss of muscle tissue and strength, sarcopenia
- Drugs can worsen this condition, for example, corticosteroids and benzodiazepines

- Orthostatic hypotension is a common condition in the elderly and can lead to injuries and lowered quality of life
- Drug treatment for cardiovascular, neurological and psychiatric disorders can cause hypotension as a side effect
- Vertigo is a disabling condition common in the elderly and a physical examination including blood pressure is necessary to determine whether orthostatic hypotension is present or not
- Commonly used drugs can be the cause of vertigo and should be considered and a re-assessment made

References

Ades PA, Ballor DL, Ashikaga T et al. (1996) Weight training improves walking endurance in healthy elderly persons. Ann Intern Med 124(6): 568–572

Andersson KE (1997) The overactive bladder: pharmacologic basis of drug treatment. Urology 50(6A Suppl): 74–84

Ashley C (2004) Renal failure – how drugs can damage the kidney. Hosp Pharmacist 11: 48–53

Bakris GL and Kern SR (1989) Renal dysfunction resulting from NSAIDs. Am Fam Physician 40(4): 199–204

Binder EF, Yarasheski KE, Steger-May K et al. (2005) Effects of progressive resistance training on body composition in frail older adults: results of a randomized, controlled trial. J Gerontol A Biol Sci Med Sci 60(11): 1425–1431

Blalock SJ, Byrd JE, Hansen RA et al. (2005) Factors associated with potentially inappropriate drug utilization in a sample of rural community-dwelling older adults. Am J Geriatr Pharmacother 3(3): 168–179

Brignole M (1998) Progressive orthostatic hypotension in the elderly. J Neurol Neurosurg Psychiatry 65: 285–289

Chapple CR (2000) Muscarinic receptor antagonists in the treatment of overactive bladder. Urology 55(5A Suppl): 33–46

Colledge NR, Wilson JA, Macintyre CC et al. (1994) The prevalence and characteristics of dizziness in an elderly community. Age Ageing 23(2): 117–120

The Consensus Committee of the American Autonomic Society and the American Academy of Neurology. (1996) Consensus statement on the definition of orthostatic hypotension, pure autonomic failure, and multiple system atrophy. Neurology 46(5): 1470

Cooper C, Atkinson EJ, Jacobsen SJ et al. (1993) Population-based study of survival after osteoporotic fractures. Am J Epidemiol 137(9): 1001–1005

Cummings SR and Melton LJ (2002) Epidemiology and outcomes of osteoporotic fractures. Lancet 359(9319): 1761–1767

Davis LE (1994) Dizziness in elderly men. J Am Geriatr Soc 42(11): 1184–1188

Doherty TJ (2003) Invited review: Aging and sarcopenia. J Appl Physiol 95(4): 1717–1727

Dutta C (1997) Significance of sarcopenia in the elderly. J Nutr 127(5 Suppl): 992S–993S

Evans WJ (1995) Effects of exercise on body composition and functional capacity of the elderly. J Gerontol A Biol Sci Med Sci 50 Spec No: 147–150

Faisal MA, Russell RM, Samloff IM et al. (1990) Helicobacter pylori infection and atrophic gastritis in the elderly. Gastroenterology 99(5): 1543–1544

Gillespie LD, Gillespie WJ, Robertson MC et al. (2009) Interventions for preventing falls in elderly people. Cochrane Database Syst Rev 15(2): CD000340

Griffin MR, Yared A, Ray WA (2000) Nonsteroidal antiinflammatory drugs and acute renal failure in elderly persons. Am J Epidemiol 151(5): 488–496

Gulmez SE, Holm A, Frederiksen H et al. (2007) Use of proton pump inhibitors and the risk of community-acquired pneumonia: a population-based case-control study. Arch Intern Med 167(9): 950–955

Hampel C, Wienhold D, Benken N et al. (1997) Prevalence and natural history of female incontinence. Eur Urol 32(Suppl 2): 3–12

Henry D, Page J, Whyte I et al. (1997) Consumption of non-steroidal anti-inflammatory drugs and the development of functional renal impairment in elderly subjects. Results of a case-control study. Br J Clin Pharmacol 44(1): 85–90

Hernández-Diaz S and García-Rodriguez LA (2000) Association between nonsteroidal anti-inflammatory drugs and upper gastrointestinal tract bleeding/perforation: an overview of epidemiologic studies published in the 1990s. Arch Intern Med 160(14): 2093–2099

Howe TE, Rochester L, Jackson A et al. (2007) Exercise for improving balance in older people. Cochrane Database Syst Rev 17(4): CD004963

Jackson S (1997) The patient with an overactive bladder – symptoms and quality-of-life issues. Urology 50(6A Suppl): 18–22

Janssen I, Shepard DS, Katzmarzyk PT et al. (2004) The healthcare costs of sarcopenia in the United States. J Am Geriatr Soc 52(1): 80–85

Johnson DA and Fennerty MB (2004) Heartburn severity underestimates erosive esophagitis severity in elderly patients with gastroesophageal reflux disease. Gastroenterology 126(3): 660–664

Jonsson R, Sixt E, Landahl S et al. (2004) Prevalence of dizziness and vertigo in an urban elderly population. J Vestib Res 14(1): 47–52

Kanis JA, Johnell O, De Laet C et al. (2002) International variations in hip fracture probabilities: implications for risk assessment. J Bone Miner Res 17(7): 1237–1244

Kemppainen H, Raiha I, Sourander L (1997) Clinical presentation of peptic ulcer in the elderly. Gerontology 43(5): 283–288

Koski K, Luukinen H, Laippala P et al. (1996) Physiological factors and medications as predictors of injurious falls by elderly people: a prospective population-based study. Age Ageing 25(1): 29–38

Kragh A (2004) [Two out of three persons living in nursing homes for the elderly are treated with at least ten different drugs. A survey of drug prescriptions in the northeastern part of Skane]. Lakartidningen 101(11): 994–996

Laine L, Ahnen D, McClain C et al. (2000) Review article: potential gastrointestinal effects of long-term acid suppression with proton pump inhibitors. Aliment Pharmacol Ther 14(6): 651–668

Leipzig RM, Cumming RG, Tinetti ME (1999a) Drugs and falls in older people: a systematic review and meta-analysis: I. Psychotropic drugs. J Am Geriatr Soc 47(1): 30–39

Leipzig RM, Cumming RG, Tinetti ME (1999b) Drugs and falls in older people: a systematic review and meta-analysis: II. Cardiac and analgesic drugs. J Am Geriatr Soc 47(1): 40–50

Manes G, Pieramico O, Uomo G et al. (2003) Relationship of sliding hiatus hernia to gastroesophageal reflux disease: a possible role for Helicobacter pylori infection? Dig Dis Sci 48(2): 303–307

Mathias CJ and Kimber JR (1998) Treatment of postural hypotension. J Neurol Neurosurg Psychiatry 65(3): 285–289

Matzke GR and Frye RF (1997) Drug administration in patients with renal insufficiency. Minimising renal and extrarenal toxicity. Drug Saf 16(3): 205–231

McConnell EJ, Tessier DJ, Wolff BG (2003) Population-based incidence of complicated diverticular disease of the sigmoid colon based on gender and age. Dis Colon Rectum 46(8): 1110–1114

Montastruc JL, Laborie I, Bagheri H, Senard JM (1997) Drug-induced orthostatic hypotension: a five-year experience in a regional pharmacovigilance centre in France. Clin Drug Invest 14(1): 61–65

Mouly S, Salom M, Tillet Y et al. (2007) Management of xerostomia in older patients: a randomised controlled trial evaluating the efficacy of a new oral lubricant solution. Drugs Aging 24(11): 957–965

Murakami T, Kawamata K, Tatekawa I et al. (1968) Gastric ulcer in elderly patients. J Gastroent 3(4): 284–285

NIH (2000) Osteoporosis prevention, diagnosis, and therapy. NIH Consensus Statement 17(1): 1–45

Oldenburg O, Kribben A, Baumgart D et al. (2002) Treatment of orthostatic hypotension. Curr Opin Pharmacol 2(6): 740–747

Payne CK (1998) Epidemiology, pathophysiology and evaluation of urinary incontinence and overactive bladder. Urology 51: 3–10

Pavri BB and Ho RT (2003) Syncope. Identifying cardiac causes in older patients. Geriatrics 58(5): 26–31

Pilotto A (1996) Helicobacter pylori infection in the elderly. Clin Geriatr 4: 53–70

Pilotto A, Franceschi M, Valerio G et al. (1999) Helicobacter pylori infection in elderly patients with peptic ulcer. Age Ageing 28(4): 412–414

Podoleanu C, Maggi R, Brignole M et al. (2006) Lower limb and abdominal compression bandages prevent progressive orthostatic hypotension in elderly persons: a randomized single-blind controlled study. J Am Coll Cardiol 48(7): 1425–1432

Ship JA, Pillemer SR, Baum BJ (2002) Xerostomia and the geriatric patient. J Am Geriatr Soc 50(3): 535–543

Talley NJ, O'Keefe EA, Zinsmeister AR et al. (1992) Prevalence of gastrointestinal symptoms in the elderly: a population-based study. Gastroenterology 102(3): 895–901

Thomson WM, Chalmers JM, Spencer AJ et al. (2000) Medication and dry mouth: findings from a cohort study of older people. J Public Health Dent 60(1): 12–20

Tinetti ME (2003) Clinical practice. Preventing falls in elderly persons. N Engl J Med 348(1): 42–49

Tramonte SM, Brand MB, Mulrow CD et al. (1997) The treatment of chronic constipation in adults. A systematic review. J Gen Intern Med 12(1): 15–24

Turner MD and Ship JA (2007) Dry mouth and its effects on the oral health of elderly people. J Am Dent Assoc 138(Suppl): 15S–20S

Uneri A and Polat S (2008) Vertigo, dizziness and imbalance in the elderly. J Laryngol Otol 122(5): 466–469

Verhaeverbeke I and Mets T (1997) Drug-induced orthostatic hypotension in the elderly: avoiding its onset. Drug Saf 17(2): 105–118

Wagner TH and Hu TW (1998) Economic costs of urinary incontinence in 1995. Urology 51(3): 355–361

WHO (1994) Assessment of fracture risk and its application to screening for postmenopausal osteoporosis. Report of a WHO Study Group. World Health Organ Tech Rep Ser 843: 1–129

Yang YX, Lewis JD, Epstein S et al. (2006) Long-term proton pump inhibitor therapy and risk of hip fracture. JAMA 296(24): 2947–2953

Zullo A, Hassan C, Campo SM et al. (2007) Bleeding peptic ulcer in the elderly: risk factors and prevention strategies. Drugs Aging 24(10): 815–828

Chapter 6
Drugs and Neuro-Psychiatric Disorders

Abstract The central nervous system (CNS) in the elderly is vulnerable. This is especially important for those old patients with diseases that affect the CNS. Cognitive impairment increases in frequency with age. Delirium is an acute disorder that affects cognition and attention. There is mostly an external cause to delirium. One common cause is drugs and before adding new drugs, withdrawal or lowering of dose of current medications should be considered. Patients with dementia may suffer from behavioural disturbances. These patients have to be treated cautiously. Affective disorders may be caused by non-psychiatric conditions. When treating affective disorders one should avoid drugs with high risk of dependence or adverse side effects such as benzodiazepines. Psychotic symptoms may be caused by drugs. When elderly patients are treated with antipsychotic drugs, doses should be as low as possible and the need should be continuously reassessed.

Keywords Cognitive impairment · Delirium · Dementia · Depression · Anxiety · Psychotic disease · Neuro-psychiatric disorders

6.1 Introduction

Aging is associated with physiologic changes in the central nervous system such as decreased cerebral blood flow and brain atrophy. This makes elderly more susceptible to adverse CNS effects from drugs. Physiological alterations that affect pharmacokinetics also contribute to the high frequency of adverse drug reactions. The increased half-time of lipid-soluble drugs e.g. long-acting benzodiazepines is an example of this.

6.2 Delirium in the Elderly

Delirium is an acute disorder that affects cognition and attention. Delirium or confusion is more frequent in advanced age. The incidence also increases with high number of medications, frailty, comobirdity and previous cognitive impairment.

P. Midlöv et al., *Drug-Related Problems in the Elderly*,
DOI 10.1007/978-90-481-2446-6_6,

Delirium is a well-known complication of hospitalisation of elderly patients. Delirium is a common condition with high prevalence in elderly in emergency departments (Elie et al. 2000). Despite the high prevalence it may be hard to detect in the emergency department and it may lengthen the need for hospital care. Delirium is a marker for emerging illness. In the intensive care unit, delirium is common and a predictor of higher mortality and longer hospital stay (Ely et al. 2004, Thomason et al. 2005). Delirium is also frequent among elderly patients with hip fractures (Furlaneto and Garcez-Leme 2006). Also for these patients, delirium is associated with increased length of hospital stay and mortality.

Elderly patients after admission to a hospital often first show mental signs and symptoms, then show behavioural disturbances (Saravay et al. 2004). Thus if early mental signs and symptoms are identified and acted on, behavioural disturbances and subsequent extended length of hospital stay may be prevented. For cognitive testing many screening instruments are available. The most widely used is probably Mini Mental State Examination (MMSE).

Delirium is a very painful condition both to the patients and to family members or personnel involved in the care of the elderly. It is also a very harmful condition. Patients with delirium have an increased risk of dementia, higher mortality and worse physical and cognitive status (Francis et al. 1990, Rockwood et al. 1999, McCusker et al. 2001). Delirium might be the only initial sign of illness such as sepsis or myocardial infarction. The underlying disease and delirium can sometimes be misdiagnosed and adequate treatment delayed. It is therefore very important to diagnose delirium and any underlying condition or external cause. Dementia has some symptoms in common with delirium but dementia is characterised by a more slow on-set and slow progression of symptoms (Table 6.1). Delirium on the other hand has a more rapid on-set and greater fluctuation in symptoms. There is mostly an external cause to delirium. In other words whereas dementia cannot be cured, delirium can by removing the external cause. Delirium is however an important marker for dementia, i.e. it increases the risk for developing dementia (Rockwood et al. 1999). Symptoms of delirium may persist up to twelve months after diagnosis (McCusker et al. 2003). Actions to identify and treat these patients should be of high priority.

Table 6.1 Differences between delirium and dementia

	Delirium	Dementia
On-set	Sudden	Often slow progressive
Time	Always fluctuation in symptoms	May have some fluctuation
Aetiology	Often an external cause	Unknown
First-line treatment	Removal of external cause is most important	Cholinesterase inhibitor

There are substantial costs due to delirium. The increased length of hospital care is obvious but also after hospital discharge the costs increase due to increased need for institutionalisation, community health care and rehabilitation.

6.2.1 Risk Factors

Delirium often has a multifactorial cause (Box 6.1). Elderly patients with severe illness or who are already cognitively impaired are vulnerable to delirium. Malnutrition or dehydration may further enhance the risk. The most common causes for delirium are drugs and diseases. Frail elderly who are vulnerable to delirium may be pushed into delirium by one dose of an inappropriate drug or by e.g. urinary retention whereas younger individuals are far more resistant.

Box 6.1 Risk factors for delirium

Multiple medications
Cognitive impairment
Dehydration or malnutrition
Severe illness
Vision impairment
Functional impairment
Sleep deprivation
Stress, e.g. transfer between care facilities

Dementia is a major risk factor for delirium. Many illnesses may increase the risk of delirium. Infections, cardiac, metabolic and of course diseases in the central nervous system may all make elderly more vulnerable to delirium. Vision impairment and functional impairment are also well-known risk factors as well as premorbid cognitive impairment (Korevaar et al. 2005, Inouye et al. 2007).

Medication is a common precipitating factor for delirium (Schor et al. 1992). Several very different medications may induce delirium in a vulnerable patient (Table 6.2). Drugs with anticholinergic effects, e.g. drugs for urinary incontinence, will in sufficiently high doses induce delirium (Karlsson 1999). Use of anticholinergic drugs increase delirium symptom severity in elderly patients with diagnosed delirium (Han et al. 2001). Benzodiazepines and antipsychotics may induce delirium. Postoperative confusion is for example more frequent in long-term benzodiazepine users (Kudoh et al. 2004). Medications that cause orthostatic reactions may in the frail elderly induce delirium. Opioids and NSAIDs are other common drugs that are known to cause delirium in the elderly. There is an overuse of psychoactive medications in elderly patients. These medications increase the risk for delirium.

Other drugs that may cause delirium are e.g., antiepileptics, digitalis, analgesics, and antidepressants. Usually the main suspects for causing drug-induced cognitive

Table 6.2 Examples of drugs that may induce delirium

Group of drugs	Examples
Antipsychotics	Thioridazine, chlorpromazine
Drugs for urinary incontinence	Oxybutynin, tolterodine
Benzodiazepines	Diazepam, flunitrazepam
Antiepileptics	Carbamazepine, phenytoin
Digitalis	Digoxin
Tricyclic antidepressive drugs	Amitriptyline, clomipramine
Analgesics	Indomethacin, dextropropoxyphene

impairment are the anticholinergic and antipsychotic drugs, and these should be the first drugs to be discontinued (Moore and O'Keeffe 1999, Alagiakrishnan and Wiens 2004). In an American study on hospitalised elderly persons five independent precipitating factors for delirium were identified: use of physical restraints, malnutrition, more than three medications added, use of bladder catheter, and any iatrogenic event (Inouye and Charpentier 1996). All acutely ill elderly patients are at risk for delirium.

6.2.2 Features of Delirium

There is most often a sudden alteration in cognition and attention. The symptoms develop during hours to days. To be able to recognise this alteration, knowledge of previous level of cognitive function is necessary. Nurses or patients' family members are important to gain this information. The delirious patients have difficulties in maintaining attention. They are easily distracted. Thinking is affected. Thoughts may be disorganised and hence, speech incoherent. The delirious patient may respond slowly, if at all. Memory is impaired. This is often more pronounced in recent memory than remote memory. Visual hallucinations are more common than auditory hallucinations. Emotional disturbances are common in delirious patients. There may be rapid shifts between different emotional states. Sleep-wake cycle disturbances are common in delirium. These include difficulty falling asleep but also a complete reversal of sleep-wake cycle. There is always a fluctuation in symptoms over time. The severity of symptoms may change very much during a 24 hours period. Psychomotor disturbances may vary from hypoactivity to hyperactivity and there is sometimes a mixed type. The patient may become restless, physical aggressive but may just as well become passive and withdrawn. Delirium with reduced motor activity may be hard to recognise. The hyperactive delirium is easier to recognise, there is however not seldom a mixed type of delirium. Patients fluctuate between hyperactive and hypoactive states.

6.2.3 Diagnosis

Delirium is a clinical diagnosis. There are no laboratory tests or radiology examinations that confirm the diagnosis. It is very important to get an adequate history from family members or staff with previous knowledge of the patient. Examination should focus not only on the mental condition but also on possible contributors to the delirium. These contributors may be a wide range of different diseases such as infections, myocardial infarction, or metabolic disturbances. The medication list should be reviewed and possible side effects considered. Adverse effects that are very rare in the younger adult should be considered as much more likely in the frail older adult. A brief cognitive screening test, i.e. Mini-Mental Status Examination, MMSE (Folstein et al. 1975) may be useful. A thorough review of the accurate medication list is mandatory in any elderly patient with delirium. Laboratory testing may be useful to differ between different predisposing and precipitating factors. Plasma-glucose and tests for renal and liver function could therefore be useful.

Dementia may be hard to differ from delirium (Table 6.1). The most important tool is a thorough medical history. Dementia has a slow progress whereas delirium is characterised by a rapid change in cognitive functions. Depression and anxiety could be mistaken for delirium, but the impaired consciousness in delirium sets it apart from affective disorders.

6.2.4 Treatment

The best thing is of course to prevent delirium. The physician should then consider the possibility of concomitant precipitating factors. Evidence on effectiveness of interventions to prevent delirium is sparse (Siddiqi et al. 2007). The use of psychoactive drugs is associated with an increased risk of delirium. Avoiding unnecessary psychoactive drugs may prevent drug-induced delirium. If delirium is at hand the aetiological factors should be identified and corrected. In many cases no other treatment is necessary. Medications with psychoactive effects should be withdrawn or given in lowered dosage. Even if aetiological factors are identified, symptomatic treatment may be needed. Nonpharmacological measures include the presence of staff or family members. A quiet environment with trained personnel is important. Personal contact is very important. Physical restraints should be avoided. There are several things that may help the patient with orientation, such as clocks and calendars. Clear signs to indicate rooms and names of staff are also useful. Hearing aids and eyeglasses are of course useful if the patient has such needs. A proper sleep environment should be enhanced since sleep deprivation may worsen the condition.

Medications may be necessary for patients with delirium especially in patients with severe behavioural disturbances and agitation. Any medications used may however be hazardous and actually lengthen the condition. A continuous reassessment of the need for theses kind of drugs should be done. Antipsychotic drugs may be needed especially if vision hallucinations and agitated behaviour are predominant. Short-acting benzodiazepines may be used for a limited time. There is no strong evidence of efficacy for antipsychotics for treatment of aggressive behaviour (Goedhard et al. 2006). Delirium is very common at the end of life. Even here delirium may be reversible. Adequate pharmacological and nonpharmacological treatment is important. Here the main purpose may not be to find the cause of delirium but to alleviate the symptoms.

6.3 Dementia

Dementia is characterised by a progressive decline in cognitive function. The prevalence of dementia increases with age. With the demographical changes, the number of patients with dementia will increase. There are three major forms of dementia; Alzheimer's disease, vascular dementia and a mixed dementia. Beside these, there are several less common subtypes of dementia.

The onset of dementia is often insidious. Patients with a slow progressive decline in cognition should be examined for possible dementia. Delirium and depression are two common diagnoses that may be hard to differ from dementia. Patients with dementia are vulnerable to medications and concomitant illnesses. Normally dementia is a slow progressive disease. Any rapid changes should be investigated. There is often an external cause such rapid change e.g. medications, change of environment, or infectious diseases.

The pharmacological treatment of Alzheimer's disease is cholinesterase inhibitor or memantine. Cholinesterase inhibitors are efficacious for mild to moderate Alzheimer's disease (Birks 2006). Adverse effects are common with these drugs e.g. nausea, bradycardia and gastro-intestinal symptoms. Often the doses are increased gradually over several weeks to minimise adverse effects. The effect of cholinesterase inhibitors is palliative, not curative. The effects and adverse effects have to be evaluated regularly. Those without any positive effect should of course not continue treatment. For patients with Alzheimer's disease a less decline in cognitive function than anticipated is an effect of great value for the patient, the family and care givers. It may result in improved quality of life and delay in nursing home admission.

Memantine is approved for treatment of moderate to severe Alzheimer's disease. It is an antagonist at glutamatergic NMDA-receptors. Memantine is well tolerated and has a small beneficial effect at six months in moderate to severe AD (McShane et al. 2006). For patients with dementia one has to be careful wit all kind of medications that may affect the central nervous system. Delirium and hallucinations are common adverse effects in patients with dementia. Agitation may be due to delirium and external causes should be ruled out before adding another psychoactive drug. Sleep disturbance is common in demented elderly patients. Sleep deprivation may in a patient with dementia induce delirium. Nonpharmacological treatment for delirium or hallucinations should be considered first.

The causes for behavioural symptoms are often multiple. Sometimes the condition is caused by a drug which then of course should be withdrawn. When antipsychotic dugs are indicated for treatment of psychosis in Alzheimer's disease atypical antipsychotics should be used in preference to typical antipsychotics (Bassiony and Lyketsos 2003). In one study low dose of risperidone had better effect on behavioural symptoms than haloperidol (De Deyn et al. 1999). Olanzapine is another atypical antipsychotic that may be used in acutely agitated patients with dementia (Meehan et al. 2002). Pharmacotherapy with antipsychotics in patients with Alzheimer's disease (AD) is however associated with high risks. In a study from 2009 there was an increased long-term risk of mortality in patients with AD who were prescribed antipsychotic medication (Ballard et al. 2009). The need for theses drugs should be reassessed.

6.4 Affective Disorders

6.4.1 Depression

Depression is common among elderly (Samuelsson et al. 2005). In a European study a prevalence of 12% was estimated among elderly living in the community (Copeland et al. 2004). Some of the symptoms in delirium are also common in depression in the elderly. Elderly have higher rates of depression but this is mostly attributable to physical health problems and related disability (Roberts et al. 1997). Depression is often underdiagnosed and inadequately treated (Bergdahl et al. 2005). Affective disorders may be caused by non-psychiatric conditions e.g. hypothyroidism, vitamin B12-deficiency and cerebrovascular insults. Other possible contributing factors are alcohol or drugs such as benzodiazepines.

The efficacy in older patients with depression has been proven not only for tricyclic antidepressants but also for selective serotonin reuptake inhibitors (SSRIs). The easy handling, the side effect profile and the safety in overdose are advantages of SSRI, which become particularly important in old age (Hegerl and Moller 2000). The anticholinergic effect is an important adverse effect that is more frequent and of greater clinical importance in the elderly taking tricyclic antidepressants. This is avoided by using SSRI as first-cline treatment in the elderly (Kompoliti and Goetz 1998). One of the SSRIs, fluoxetine, has a long half-life in older adults and therefore citalopram, sertraline or paroxetine are preferred in the elderly.

Selective serotonin re-uptake inhibitors (SSRI) are often effective in treating elderly patients with depression. There is however a lack of studies on treatment of late life depression (Freudenstein et al. 2001). When treating with SSRIs doses should be low and then titrated up. One should be aware of possible withdrawal syndrome when these drugs are discontinued. There are also important interactions for SSRI. Both with drugs i.e. aspirin (acetylsalisylic acid) increased risk of gastrointestinal bleeding as well as in certain concomitant diseases, i.e. SSRI may increase the risk of epileptic seizures. Tricyclic antidepressants as well as SSRIs also increase the risk for falls among nursing home residents (Thapa et al. 1998). There is a dose-response relation. When insufficient effect with SSRIs, mirtazapine, venlafaxine and for severe depressions treatment with electroconvulsive therapy (ECT) may be considered. Older drugs such as tricyclic antidepressants may be used but they are generally less well tolerated.

Lithium is commonly used for bipolar affective disorders. Lithium however has a narrow therapeutic index and high risk for toxicity (Groleau 1994). The use of loop diuretics or ACE-inhibitors significantly increases the risk of hospitalisation for lithium toxicity in the elderly (Juurlink et al. 2004). Treatment of elderly patients with lithium should be thoroughly monitored.

6.4.2 Anxiety

Anxiety is common among the elderly but the literature regarding the assessment, diagnosis, and treatment of these illnesses in older individuals is sparse (Blazer 1997). Most often anxiety does not present for the first time in late life. If that is the case one should suspect an underlying condition or other external cause. These causes could be medications such as digitalis, antipsychotics but also conditions as anaemia, chronic obstructive lung disease with hypoxia or myocardial infarction.

When treating anxiety one should of course first treat any reversible medical condition. When pharmacological treatment is necessary SSRI is most often drug of choice. Selective serotonin reuptake inhibitors are both effective and safe. Benzodiazepines that have been widely used are drugs with a relative high risk of adverse effects (see Chapter 4). Risks for dependence and abuse must always be considered for benzodiazepines.

6.5 Psychotic Disease

The prevalence of psychotic symptoms has been estimated to 5–6% among elderly (Henderson et al. 1998). One important risk factor for psychotic symptoms in the elderly is cognitive impairment. Psychotic symptoms may be more common among the very old (Ostling et al. 2007). The elderly may be reluctant to report psychotic symptoms and therefore a thorough history from older patients but also from their family members is important. A presentation of psychotic symptoms in a patient with no previous history of psychotic disease should make the physician consider medications or an underlying medical condition as potential causes. As mentioned above patients with delirium or dementia often have psychotic symptoms. Several medications may cause the psychotic symptoms. Opiates, anticholinergic drugs and dopaminergic drugs (for Parkinson's disease) may cause these symptoms.

The prevalence rates of schizophrenia are lower in old age than in younger age groups (Copeland et al. 1998). The incidence of Alzheimer's disease with psychosis is much more frequent than the incidence of schizophrenia in old age (Jeste and Finkel 2000). For the frail Alzheimer's patients, medications may induce or aggravate the symptoms.

For psychotic elderly first step is to remove any possible contributor. When the symptoms remain, antipsychotics should be considered. Doses should stay as low as possible. Many antipsychotics have sedating as well as extrapyramidal side effects. A very troublesome problem in the elderly is tardive dyskinesia. There may also be effects on the cardiovascular system such as orthostatic reactions. There is no evidence that benzodiazepines with or without antipsychotic drugs should be used for acute psychosis (Gillies et al. 2005).

6.6 Conclusions

- Delirium is a severe condition that in the elderly often is caused by drugs
- Delirium and hallucinations are common adverse effects in patients with dementia
- Anticholinergic effect is an important adverse effect that is frequent in the elderly taking tricyclic antidepressants
- Alzheimer's disease with psychosis is much more frequent than the incidence of schizophrenia in old age

References

Alagiakrishnan K and Wiens CA (2004) An approach to drug induced delirium in the elderly. Postgrad Med J 80(945): 388–393

Ballard C, Hanney ML, Theodoulou M et al. (2009) The dementia antipsychotic withdrawal trial (DART-AD): long-term follow-up of a randomised placebo-controlled trial. The Lancet Neurology DOI:10.1016/S1474-4422(08)70295-3

Bassiony MM and Lyketsos CG (2003) Delusions and hallucinations in Alzheimer's disease: review of the brain decade. Psychosomatics 44 (5): 388–401

Bergdahl E, Gustavsson JM, Kallin K et al. (2005) Depression among the oldest old: the Umea 85+ study. Int Psychogeriatr 17 (4): 557–575

Birks J (2006) Cholinesterase inhibitors for Alzheimer's disease. Cochrane Database Syst Rev 25 (1): CD005593

Blazer DG (1997) Generalized anxiety disorder and panic disorder in the elderly: a review. Harv Rev Psychiatry 5 (1): 18–27

Copeland JR, Beekman AT, Braam AW et al. (2004) Depression among older people in Europe: the EURODEP studies. World Psychiatry 3 (1): 45–49

Copeland JR, Dewey ME, Scott A et al. (1998) Schizophrenia and delusional disorder in older age: community prevalence, incidence, comorbidity, and outcome. Schizophr Bull 24 (1): 153–161

De Deyn PP, Rabheru K, Rasmussen A et al. (1999) A randomized trial of risperidone, placebo, and haloperidol for behavioral symptoms of dementia. Neurology 53(5): 946–955

Elie M, Rousseau F, Cole M et al. (2000) Prevalence and detection of delirium in elderly emergency department patients. Cmaj 163(8): 977–981

Ely EW, Shintani A, Truman B et al. (2004) Delirium as a predictor of mortality in mechanically ventilated patients in the intensive care unit. JAMA 291 (14): 1753–1762

Folstein MF, Folstein SE, McHugh PR (1975) "Mini-mental state". A practical method for grading the cognitive state of patients for the clinician. J Psychiatr Res 12 (3): 189–198

Francis J, Martin D, Kapoor WN (1990) A prospective study of delirium in hospitalized elderly. JAMA 263 (8): 1097–1101

Freudenstein U, Jagger C, Arthur A et al. (2001) Treatments for late life depression in primary care–a systematic review. Fam Pract 18 (3): 321–327

Furlaneto ME and Garcez-Leme LE (2006) Delirium in elderly individuals with hip fracture: causes, incidence, prevalence, and risk factors. Clinics 61 (1): 35–40

Gillies D, Beck A, McCloud A et al. (2005) Benzodiazepines alone or in combination with antipsychotic drugs for acute psychosis. Cochrane Database Syst Rev 19 (4): CD003079

Goedhard LE, Stolker JJ, Heerdink ER et al. (2006) Pharmacotherapy for the treatment of aggressive behavior in general adult psychiatry: A systematic review. J Clin Psychiatry 67 (7): 1013–1024

Groleau G (1994) Lithium toxicity. Emerg Med Clin North Am 12 (2): 511–531

Han L, McCusker J, Cole M et al. (2001) Use of medications with anticholinergic effect predicts clinical severity of delirium symptoms in older medical inpatients. Arch Intern Med 161 (8): 1099–1105

Hegerl U and Moller HJ (2000) [Pharmacotherapy of depression in the elderly]. Nervenarzt 71 (1): 1–8

Henderson AS, Korten AE, Levings C et al. (1998) Psychotic symptoms in the elderly: a prospective study in a population sample. Int J Geriatr Psychiatry 13 (7): 484–492

Inouye SK and Charpentier PA (1996) Precipitating factors for delirium in hospitalized elderly persons. Predictive model and interrelationship with baseline vulnerability. JAMA 275 (11): 852–857

Inouye SK, Zhang Y, Jones RN et al. (2007) Risk factors for delirium at discharge: development and validation of a predictive model. Arch Intern Med 167 (13): 1406–1413

Jeste DV and Finkel SI (2000) Psychosis of Alzheimer's disease and related dementias. Diagnostic criteria for a distinct syndrome. Am J Geriatr Psychiatry 8 (1): 29–34

Juurlink DN, Mamdani MM, Kopp A et al. (2004) Drug-induced lithium toxicity in the elderly: a population-based study. J Am Geriatr Soc 52 (5): 794–798

Karlsson I (1999) Drugs that induce delirium. Dement Geriatr Cogn Disord 10 (5): 412–415

Kompoliti K and Goetz CG (1998) Neuropharmacology in the elderly. Neurol Clin 16 (3): 599–610

Korevaar JC, van Munster BC, de Rooij SE (2005) Risk factors for delirium in acutely admitted elderly patients: a prospective cohort study. BMC Geriatr 5: 6

Kudoh A, Takase H, Takahira Y et al. (2004) Postoperative confusion increases in elderly long-term benzodiazepine users. Anesth Analg 99 (6): 1674–1678

McCusker J, Cole M, Dendukuri N et al. (2001) Delirium in older medical inpatients and subsequent cognitive and functional status: a prospective study. Cmaj 165 (5): 575–583

McCusker J, Cole M, Dendukuri N et al. (2003) The course of delirium in older medical inpatients: a prospective study. J Gen Intern Med 18 (9): 696–704

McShane R, Areosa Sastre A, Minakaran N (2006) Memantine for dementia. Cochrane Database Syst Rev 19 (2): CD003154

Meehan KM, Wang H, David SR et al. (2002) Comparison of rapidly acting intramuscular olanzapine, lorazepam, and placebo: a double-blind, randomized study in acutely agitated patients with dementia. Neuropsychopharmacology 26 (4): 494–504

Moore AR and O'Keeffe ST (1999) Drug-induced cognitive impairment in the elderly. Drugs Aging 15 (1): 15–28

Ostling S, Borjesson-Hanson A, Skoog I (2007) Psychotic symptoms and paranoid ideation in a population-based sample of 95-year-olds. Am J Geriatr Psychiatry 15 (12): 999–1004

Roberts RE, Kaplan GA, Shema SJ et al. (1997) Does growing old increase the risk for depression? Am J Psychiatry 154 (10): 1384–1390

Rockwood K, Cosway S, Carver D et al. (1999) The risk of dementia and death after delirium. Age Ageing 28 (6): 551–556

Samuelsson G, McCamish-Svensson C, Hagberg B et al. (2005) Incidence and risk factors for depression and anxiety disorders: results from a 34-year longitudinal Swedish cohort study. Aging Ment Health 9 (6): 571–575

Saravay SM, Kaplowitz M, Kurek J et al. (2004) How do delirium and dementia increase length of stay of elderly general medical inpatients? Psychosomatics 45 (3): 235–242

Schor JD, Levkoff SE, Lipsitz LA et al. (1992) Risk factors for delirium in hospitalized elderly. JAMA 267 (6): 827–831

Siddiqi N, Stockdale R, Britton AM et al. (2007) Interventions for preventing delirium in hospitalised patients. Cochrane Database Syst Rev 18 (2): CD005563

Thapa PB, Gideon P, Cost TW et al. (1998) Antidepressants and the risk of falls among nursing home residents. N Engl J Med 339 (13): 875–882

Thomason JW, Shintani A, Peterson JF et al. (2005) Intensive care unit delirium is an independent predictor of longer hospital stay: a prospective analysis of 261 non-ventilated patients. Crit Care 9 (4): R375–R381

Chapter 7
Errors, Problems, Events and Reactions on Medication

Abstract Humans are prone to errors, e.g. almost 100,000 Americans die each year due to mistakes in medical care. Drug-related problems can occur in all steps in the drug therapy process. This can be caused by various types of medication errors including prescribing, dispensing, labelling, administration, handling, documentation, information, communication, and follow-up, and can result in patient injuries. Medication errors are common although few results in adverse drug events. The elderly have higher risks due to several reasons. In this chapter we present definitions and problems as a base for practical models, interventions, and improvements which are presented in later chapters.

Keywords Medication errors · Drug-related problems · Adverse drug event · Adverse drug reaction · Risk patients

7.1 Introduction

Real or potential drug-related problems (DRP) can occur in all steps from prescribing to use and follow up on effects. This can be caused by a medication error, made by health-care professionals, by the patient and in the interaction and communication between those. There can be patient injuries (adverse drug events, ADE) from medications errors or other reasons such as, adverse drug reactions (ADR). An ADR causing injury for the patient is an ADE. ADE can also result from low or no treatment efficacy or no or wrong treatment of the condition (extrinsic DRP, a medication error). Medication errors are common although few results in intrinsic DRPs and ADE. In one inpatient study the frequency of medication errors were 5.3 per 100 medication orders compared to 0.25 for ADE (Bates et al. 1995). In a more recent study the error rate was 19 per 100 doses and 7% of the errors were judged as potential adverse drug events (Barker et al. 2002). A summary of the described relationships is presented in Fig. 7.1.

DOI 10.1007/978-90-481-2446-6_7,

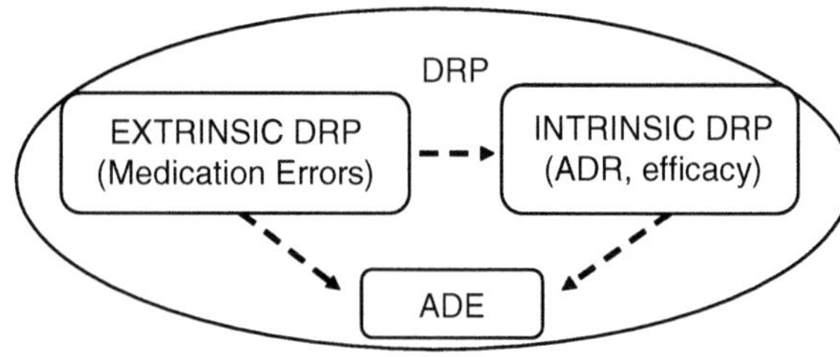

Fig. 7.1 Relationship between Drug-related Problems (DRP), Adverse Drug Reaction (ADR), and Adverse Drug Event (ADE). The definitions of extrinsic and intrinsic DRPs have been adapted from van den Bent (2002)

7.2 Medication Errors

Medication error has been defined as "Any error in the process of prescribing, dispensing, or administering a drug, whether there are adverse consequences or not" (Leape 1995). The incidence of medication errors in medical wards at a US tertiary care hospital has been described from a pioneer study (Bates et al. 1995). Of 10,070 medication orders 530 medication errors were identified, for a mean 0.3 medication errors per patient-day, or 1.4 per admission. 53% involved at least one missing dose of medication, 15% involved other dose errors, 8% frequency errors, and 5% route errors. Error rates in observational studies of the medication administration process have been summarised (Flynn and Barker 2006). Because of differences in error category definitions as methods they state that caution should be used in comparisons. Errors, excluding wrong-time errors, have been estimated to occur at a rate of about one per patient per day. With unit dose systems the error rate decreased to two to three per patient per week. Also studies on pharmacy dispensing errors were reviewed. "Picking-errors" in the in-patient setting ranged from 0.04% to 2.9%. The prescription filling operations had an error rate from 1% to 24%. The rate of errors that could potentially have harmed the patients was 1.5–4%.

The National Coordinating Council for Medication Error Reporting and Prevention (NCC MERP) mission is to maximise the safe use of medications and to increase awareness of medication errors through open communication, increased reporting and promotion of medication error prevention strategies. On their homepage (NCC-MERP 2008) recommendations, tools (trigger tools see Chapter 10) and other support are available for research and practice improvement. Methods for detecting errors include anonymous self reports, incident reports, critical incident technique, chart review, computerised monitoring and direct observation.

Also the Institute for Safe Medication Practices (ISMP) deserves great attention (ISMP 2008). ISMP is a non-profit organisation educating the health care community and consumers on safe medication practices. The group has more than 30 years of experience in the field and the book Medication Errors edited by Michael Cohen (Cohen 2006) is probably the most extensive and updated in the field. Very important aspects and priorities like root case analysis, drug nomenclature and similar names, unsafe drug packaging, unsafe labelling and advertising, unsafe abbreviations and symbols, application of technology for error prevention, and much more are presented. For a hospital a starting point can be as described in Box 7.1.

Box 7.1 Starting point for reducing medication errors in hospitals

- Systematic, simple and practice oriented instructions for medication use and handling at each ward.
- Restricted formulary at each ward with well known medications. Supported with routines and standardized stock ordering and prescribing modules.
- Special attention on high-alert medications, including identification, labelling and education.
- Follow-up on medication errors, including knowledge of routines, incidence reporting, root case analysis etc.
- Medication Reconciliation (Chapter 10)

It should be stated that medication errors can be made by health care professionals, but also by the patient, or a combination of both as highlighted in Table 7.1. Different aspects of these errors, consequences and interventions for improvement are presented in this book

Table 7.1 Reasons for medication errors based on responsibilities

Health care professional	Shared	Patient/spouse/ relative
Prescribing	Communication	Handling
Dispensing	Concordance	Administration
Labelling	Documentation	Compliance
Administration	Follow-up	Information
Handling		
Documentation		
Information		

7.2.1 To Err is Human

In 1999, the Institute of Medicine (IOM) estimate that 48,000–98,000 Americans die each year in the hospital because of mistakes and oversights in medical care (Kohn et al. 1999). The report, To Err Is Human: Building a Safer Health Care System, states the fact that humans are prone to error. Therefore systems in health care cannot depend on human perfection. Like in airlines and nuclear power industry we need highly safe operations and we must take into account human mistakes in training, systems design, and organisation management. The IOM report raised public and professional awareness of the need for changing the health care system and make recommendations on leadership and knowledge, identifying and learning from errors, setting performance standards and expectations for safety, implementing safety systems in health care organisations.

7.2.2 5 Million Live Campaign

The Institute for Healthcare Improvement (IHI) (IHI 2008) launched a national American campaign for improvement and five years after the IOM report Leape and Berwick summarise what has happened, analysed the reasons why improvement has not been greater, and made recommendations for what needs to be accomplished to realise the IOM's vision (Leape and Berwick 2005). After that IHI has launched a new campaign (5 Million lives) and added intervention targets as presented in Box 7.2(IHI 2008). The specific drug-related problems and interventions are market in bold and will be highlighted below.

Box 7.2 Campaign interventions from IHI

The six interventions from the 100,000 Lives Campaign

- Deploy Rapid Response Teams. . .at the first sign of patient decline
- Deliver Reliable, Evidence-Based Care for Acute Myocardial Infarction. . .to prevent deaths from heart attack
- Prevent Adverse Drug Events (**ADEs**). . .by implementing **medication reconciliation**
- Prevent Central Line Infections. . .by implementing a series of interdependent, scientifically grounded steps
- Prevent Surgical Site Infections. . .by reliably delivering the correct perioperative antibiotics at the proper time
- Prevent Ventilator-Associated Pneumonia. . .by implementing a series of interdependent, scientifically grounded steps

New interventions targeted at harm

- Prevent Harm from **High-Alert Medications**. . . starting with a focus on anticoagulants, sedatives, narcotics, and insulin
- Reduce Surgical Complications. . . by reliably implementing all of the changes in care recommended by SCIP, the Surgical Care Improvement Project (www.medqic.org/scip)
- Prevent Pressure Ulcers. . . by reliably using science-based guidelines for their prevention
- Reduce Methicillin-Resistant Staphylococcus aureus (MRSA) infection. . .by reliably implementing scientifically proven infection control practices
- Deliver Reliable, Evidence-Based Care for Congestive Heart Failure. . . to avoid readmissions

- Get Boards on Board ... by defining and spreading the best-known leveraged processes for hospital Boards of Directors, so that they can become far more effective in accelerating organizational progress toward safe care.

Similar national campaigns, action-planes or activities have followed in other countries. A European Network for Patient Safety (EUNetPaS) was launched in 2008 (EUNet-PaS 2008). The project, aims to establish an umbrella network of all 27 EU Member States and EU stake holders to encourage and enhance collaboration in the field of Patient Safety. It focuses on five key patient safety topic areas; promoting a culture of patient safety; structuring education and training; proposal of a core European curricula higher education; implementing reporting and learning systems; pilot implementation of medication safety. The latter has full focus on improving medication safety in hospitals by identifying good practices, translating them into tools and testing these tools in selected hospitals.

7.3 Drug-Related Problems

Drug-related problems can be defined as "Any undesirable event experienced by the patient that involves or is suspected to involve drug therapy and that actually or potentially interferes with a desired patient outcome" (Strand et al.1990). This is a vital component of Pharmaceutical Care and Clinical Pharmacy and will be described more in detail in another chapter. It should however be noted that there are several definitions and classification systems for DRPs. A literature review (van Mil et al. 2004) identified fourteen classifications and their critical elements. In the presented definition a potential problem is a DRP but this is not the case in all definitions and classifications. This is also the case for unavoidable adverse drug reactions (e.g. with cytotoxic agents).

7.4 Adverse Drug Events

An adverse drug event (ADE) can be defined as "An injury related to the use of a drug, although the causality of this relationship may not be proven" (Leape 1995). Medications are the most frequent cause of adverse event. In a review it was reported that ADEs are common in most clinical settings included adult inpatients (reported incidences of 6.5%), adult outpatients (27.4%), and a paediatric inpatients (2.3%) (Morimoto et al. 2004). No data on the elderly was reported but it is probably even higher than in adult settings.

7.5 Adverse Drug Reactions

An adverse drug reaction is defined by WHO as "A response to a drug which is noxious and unintended, and which occurs at doses normally used in man for the prophylaxis, diagnosis, or therapy of disease, or for the modification of physiological function" (WHO 1995). This basic definition includes all doses prescribed clinically, but is intended to exclude accidental or deliberate overdose. As described previously ADRs in the elderly is much more common than reported in clinical trials, it is also often (up to 90%) preventable (Beijer et al. 2002). The background for this is presented in Chapter 2.

7.5.1 WHO Programme for International Drug Monitoring

The programme provides a forum for WHO member states to collaborate in the monitoring of drug safety. Within the programme, individual case reports of suspected adverse drug reactions are collected and stored in a common database, presently containing over 3.7 million case reports. In each of the countries participating in the programme, the government has designated a national centre for pharmacovigilance (WHO-UMC 2008).

The programme consists of a network of the national centres, WHO headquarters, Geneva and the WHO Collaborating Centre for International Drug Monitoring, the Uppsala Monitoring Centre, in Uppsala, Sweden. As of July 2008, 84 countries had joined the programme, and in addition, 33 countries were considered associate members.

7.5.2 Pharmacovigilance and Reporting

Pharmacovigilance is described as "The science and activities relating to the detection, assessment, understanding and prevention of adverse effects or any other drug-related problems" (WHO 2002). Reporting adverse drug reactions in clinical practice and in clinical trials is mandatory and part of pharmacovigilanc activities. The spontaneous reporting is mainly focusing on serious and new events. Prescribers, pharmacists, nurses and also patients can be reporters depending on national regulations. This reporting is the base for information on adverse drug reactions in Summaries of Products Characteristics (SPC) produced by Medication Authorities, which is the base for further information. The recommended standard categories of frequency reporting (WHO 1995) are shown in Box 7.3.

Box 7.3 Frequency reporting of adverse drug reactions

Very common	> 1/10	(> 10%)
Common(frequent)	> 1/100 and < 1/10	(> 1% and < 10%)
Uncommon (infrequent)	> 1/1,000 and < 1/100	(> 0,1% and < 1%)
Rare	> 1/10,000 and < 1,000	(> 0,01% and < 0,1%)
Very rare	< 1/10,000	(< 0,01%)

7.6 Risk Medications

Prevent harm from high-alert medications starting with a focus on anticoagulants, sedatives, narcotics, and insulin is one of the primary goals of the 5 Million Lives Campaign presented above. On their homepage (IHI 2008) getting started kits, mentor hospitals, and measurement information forms are provided. Based on error reports submitted to a program the Institute for Safe Medication Practices (ISMP) has produced a list of High-Alert Medications (ISMP 2008). The list (Box 7.4) includes drugs that bear a heightened risk of causing significant patient harm when they are used in error. ISMP suggest strategies to special safeguards to reduce the risk of errors including restricted use; high access to information when used; using auxiliary labels and automated alerts; standardized ordering, storage, preparation, and administration; and employing redundancies such as automated or independent double-checks when necessary.

Box 7.4 Some high alert medication relevant for use in the elderly (adopted from ISMP 2008). For a complete list consult ISMP 2008

Drug classes/categories (examples)

- Adrenergic agonists IV (epinephrine, phenylephrine)
- Adrenergic antagonists IV (propranolol, methoprolol)
- Anesthetics general, inhaled, IV (propofol, ketamine)
- Antiarrytmics IV (lidocaine, amidarone)
- Antitrombotics and Anticoagulants (warfarin, heparin, LMWH, Factor Xa inhibitors, direct trombin inhibitors, thrombolytics, and glycoprotein inhibitors)
- Cardioplegic solutions
- Chemotherapeutic agents, parenteral and IV
- Dextrose hypertonic, 20% or greater
- Dialysis solutions
- Epidural and intrathecal medications
- Hypoglycemics, oral
- Inotropics IV (digoxin, milrinone)
- Liposomal forms of drugs (amfotericin B)
- Moderate sedation agents IV (midazolam)
- Narcotics/opiates IV, transdermal, oral
- Neuromuscular blockers (succinylcholine,rocuronium)
- Radiocontrast agents IV
- Total parental nutrition solutions

Specific drugs

- Colchicin injection
- Epoprostenol (Flolan) IV
- Insulin subcutaneous and IV
- Magnesium sulfate injection
- Methotrexate oral non-oncology use
- Nitroprusside sodium for injection
- Potassium chloride for injection concentrate
- Potassium phosphates injection
- Sodium chloride for injection hypertonic (>0.9%)
- Sterile water for injection and irrigation (excl pour bottles) in containers of 100 ml or more.

7.7 Risk Patients—The Elderly

A significant prevalence of ADRs was found among hospitalised elderly people in Brazil (Passarelli et al. 2005). The risk factors associated with ADRs included use of drugs considered to be inappropriate, number of previous diagnoses, and number of administered drugs. More appropriate drug prescription was stated to avoid part of this burden of disease by minimising preventable ADRs. They also conclude that the elderly of course have a higher risk to suffer from harm from these high-alert medications since the frequency of exposure and the risk of adverse events is higher.

Several of the individual problems and risks increasing and cumulating the risk for morbidity and mortality in the elderly are presented in this book. Each of them is presented in more detail elsewhere. Special attention should be given to patients with severe diseases, polypharmacy, high-alert medications, several prescribers, several acute hospital admissions, and low compliance. It is important to understand that the problems and risks are interconnected. One problem lead to another in a cascade, where the net benefit to harm relation, might be negative.

Polypharmacy is often a consequence of the cascade of problems. A literature review found that polypharmacy continues to increase and is a known risk factor for important morbidity and mortality (Hajjar et al. 2007). The reviewers states that "many studies have found that various numbers of medications are associated with negative health outcomes, but more research is needed to further delineate the consequences associated with unnecessary drug use in elderly patients. Health care professionals should be aware of the risks and fully evaluate all medications at each patient visit to prevent polypharmacy from occurring".

7.8 Conclusions

- Since the elderly use many drugs they are at high risk for medication errors and also for medication injuries, causing waste of resources and human suffering
- Many international organisations have focused on prevention of errors and harm and have identified problems and developed tools and campaigns for awareness and improvement
- There is a mutual responsibility between the health care professionals and patients to identify, resolve and prevent drug-related problems

References

Barker KN, Flynn EA, Pepper GA, Bates DW, Mikeal RL (2002) Medication errors observed in 36 health care facilities. Arch Intern Med 162: 1897–1903

Bates DW, Boyle DL, Vander Vliet MB, Schneider J, Leape L (1995) Relationship between medication errors and adverse drug events. J Gen Intern Med 10: 199–205

Cohen MR (ed) (2006) Medication errors. American Pharmaceutical Association, Washington, DC

EUNet-PaS (2008) The European Network for Patient Safety. http://www.eunetpas.eu. Cited 30 Dec 2008

Flynn EA and Barker KN (2006) Medication errors research. In: Cohen MR (ed) Medication errors. American Pharmaceutical Association, Washington, DC

Hajjar ER, Cafiero AC, Hanlon JT (2007) Polypharmacy in elderly patients. Am J Geriatr Pharmacother 5: 345–351

Kohn LT, Corrigan JM, Donaldson MS (eds) (1999) To err is human: Building a safer health system. National Academies Press, Washington, DC

IHI (2008) Institute for health care improvement. Protecting 5 million lives from harm. http://www.ihi.org/IHI/Programs/Campaign/Campaign.htm?TabId=1. Cited 30 Dec 2008

ISMP (2008) Institute for safe medication practices. ISMP list of High-Alert Medications) http://www.ismp.org/Tools/highalertmedications.pdf. Cited 30 Dec 2008

Leape LL and Berwick DM (2005) Five years after to err is human: What have we learned? JAMA 293: 2384–2390

Leape LL (1995) Preventing adverse drug events. Am J Health Syst Pharm 52: 379–382

Morimoto T, Gandhi TK, Fiskio JM, Seger AC, So JW, Cook EF, Fukui T, Bates DW (2004) An evaluation of risk factors for adverse drug events associated with angiotensin-converting enzyme inhibitors. J Eval Clin Pract 10: 499–509

NCC-MERP (2008) The National Coordinating Council for Medication Error Reporting and Prevention. http://www.nccmerp.org. Cited 30 Dec 2008

Passarelli MC, Jacob-Filho W, Figueras A (2005) Adverse drug reactions in an elderly hospitalised population: inappropriate prescription is a leading cause. Drugs Aging 22: 767–777

Strand LM, Morley PC, Cipolle RJ, Ramsey R, Lamsam GD (1990) Drug-related problems: their structure and function. DICP 24: 1093–1097

van den Bent PMLA (2002) Drug safety in hospitalised patients. Dissertation, University of Enschede, The Netherlands

van Mil JW, Westerlund LO, Hersberger KE, Schaefer MA (2004) Drug-related problem classification systems. Ann Pharmacother 38: 859–867

WHO (1972) World Health Organisation. Technical support series no 498

WHO (1995) Good safety information practices. In: Guidelines for preparing core clinical safety information on drugs-Report of CIOMS working group III. World Health Organisation, Geneva, Switzerland

WHO (2002) The Importance of Pharmacovigilance. World Health Organisation, Geneva, Switzerland

WHO-UMC (2008) WHO Collaborating Centre for International Drug Monitoring. Uppsala Monitoring Centre. http://www.who-umc.org. Cited 30 Dec 2008

Chapter 8
Practical Problems Related to the Patients Medication Intake

Abstract Why do patients refer to medications as the little white pill or the pink capsule? Strange or confusing names are problematic especially if you are old and have many medications. Other potential practical medication problems in the elderly including problems to remember, to swallow, practical handling, food- and drug-interactions, short use-before date are listed and described in this chapter. Possible solutions are also presented. For patient safety and for cost-effective care it's very important to identify and solve these problems for the individual patient. A systematic model for this is presented in Chapter 10.

Keywords Practical problems · Generic drug · Analogue drug · Medication intake · Food interactions

8.1 Confusing Names

A drug includes various ingredients dependent on the therapeutic effects and on the route for administration. A tablet or a capsule for oral administration includes normally one active ingredient and inactive ingredients (excipients or constituents) such as bulk-agents (i.e. lactose) to get the right size, and glidant/anti-adherent agents (i.e. magnesium stearate) for easier manufacturing.

An active ingredient with potential as a drug gets a substance name early in the development (i.e. omeprazole). When first approved for use the drug gets a trade name suggested by the applicant (The pharmaceutical company). In the omeprazole case Losec/Prilosec is the original and patented trade name. When the patent time has passed other pharmaceutical companies can manufacture and sell omeprazole using their own name. Often this name is the substance name followed by the company name (i.e. Omeprazole XPharma). Nowadays the original trade name is normally identical within the European Union and also in the United States.

To further explore the problems with trade names of drugs some examples are given. The basis for this is that trade names of drugs can be a combination of original trade name, generic trade name, active ingredient (substance name, generic name) plus company name, formulation and indication for use. The Institute for Safe Medication Practices has produced a list of confused drug names (ISMP 2005).

P. Midlöv et.al., *Drug-Related Problems in the Elderly*,
DOI 10.1007/978-90-481-2446-6_8,

8.1.1 Original and Generic Drugs

For first approval of a new active ingredient (resulting in the original patented trade name) extensive documentation of chemical, pharmaceutical, pharmacological and clinical properties and effects is required by the authorities (ICH 2008, EU 2001). After approximately ten years of market exclusivity other companies can produce and market copies of the original drug, generic medicinal product, if patent on the substance and formulation has expired. A generic medicinal product is defined as a medicinal product that has the same qualitative and quantitative composition in active substances and the same pharmaceutical form as the reference medicinal product and whose bioequivalence (with the reference medicinal product) has been demonstrated with appropriate bioavailability studies (EU 2001 specific Article 10 (2)(b)). Some minor deviations in salts, isomers etcetera are accepted. Guidance for investigation on bioavailability and bioequivalence are available (CPMP 2000). A short summary of bioequivalence testing is provided in Box 8.1.

Box 8.1 Bioequivalence testing (Christians et al. 2000)

Aim: Show that two pharmaceutical products have the same pharmacokinetic properties and the same bioavailability.
Study design; Randomised two period cross-over, 12–36 healthy volunteers.
Comparisons: Area under the curve (AUC), Maximum concentration (Cmax) and time to Cmax (Tmax)
Bioequivalence: 90% Confidence interval (test/ref) within $\pm$20% (0.8–1.25)
Comment. The studies summarise intra- and inter- individual variability.

The company that applies for approval of the generic product must present full chemical and pharmaceutical documentation. If the new product does not fall within the definition of a generic medicinal product compared to the reference product the results of the appropriate pre-clinical tests or clinical trials should be provided (EU 2001 specific Article 10 (3)). It should be noted that the pharmaceutical and chemical quality is strictly regulated and includes all medications.

Normally the price is much decreased for generic copies and the economic benefit from substitution can be large for the patient and very large for the society. Different rules for substitution on pharmacies are applied in different countries. Also for some medications with narrow therapeutic indices and used for critical conditions (i.e. medications for Epilepsy and organ transplantations) the products are not exchangeable (at pharmacies) on the patient level. Some examples of original and generic products and names are given in Table 8.1.

Table 8.1 Examples of original and generic medicinal products

Product name	Comment
Losec, Prilosec Losec MUPS, Prilosec MUPS	All products include omeprazole as active ingredient. Losec and Prilosec are original medicinal products in Europe and USA respectively. MUPS (Multi Unit Pellet System) is also an original trade name and drug formulation
Omeprazole XPharma.	Omeprazole XPharma is a generic product which is bioequivalent to the original products, MUPS included.
Losec MUPS XPharma	Losec MUPS XPharma is identical to the original and parallel imported by XPharma
Tegretol, Tegretol Retard, Hermolepsin and Hermolepsin Retard	All products have carbamazepine as active ingredients. Retard is slow release formulations. The products have different pharmacokinetics and are not bioequivalent.
Lamictal and Lamotrigine X Pharma	Both products have lamotrigine as active ingredients. Lamotrigine is a generic copy of Lamictal but not exchangeable.

It should be noted that there might also be small differences (similar to differences for generic products) between different batches of original and generic products. However this potential differences and differences between original and generic products are very small compared to other patient factors affecting the pharmacokinetics and pharmacodynamics in an individual patient. This includes disease states, genetic and environment factors, other medication etcetera. This are described more in detail in Chapter 2.

8.1.2 Parallel Imported Drugs

The Pharmaceutical companies want to maximise there profit on drugs. To do this there might be price differences between markets and countries. In this case another pharmaceutical company can buy the drug in one country and sell it in another. Despite the costs for re-labelling and repacking there might be a profit for the parallel importing company. An example is shown in Table 8.1.

8.1.3 Analogue Drugs

Analogue drugs (me-too drugs) is structurally very similar to already known drugs. These drugs are developed as original products but are really medically equivalent products with different active ingredients and the same mode of action to new, interesting and potentially very profitable products. Lanzoprazole, pantoprazole, and esomeprazole are analogue products to the first proton pump inhibitor (PPI) on the market, omeprazole (Losec). These products can differ in pharmacological aspects (potency, dosing etcetera) and also often in the documentation in specific patient populations. The value of these products for society and for the companies on a long term perspective is debated.

8.1.4 Other Product Names

Combinations of active ingredients, specific pharmaceutical formulations, specific use, and company names can be included in the product name. Examples of this are shown in Table 8.2. This combinations and mixes of names can be very complicated and disturbing for the health-care and for the patients, especially for the elderly. It not easy to know what is important. Is ZOC a company or a pharmaceutical formulation changing the dosing schedule? Patient safety in the reconciliation of medicines as described in Chapter 10 is very important and must not be neglected.

Table 8.2 Examples of drug names based on product, substance, and company names, and also on formulations, and specific use

Product name	Comment
Renitec, Renitec Comp, Enalapril XPharma, Enalapril Comp XPharma, Renitec Comp XPharma	All products have enalapril as active ingredients. Comp means that the product is a combination with a diuretic. Enalapril Comp XPharma is a generic copy and Renitec Comp XPharma is a parallel imported product
Seloken, Seloken ZOC	Both products have metoprolol as active ingredient. ZOC is a slow release formulation.
Emconcor, Emconcor CHF, Bisoprolol XPharma.	All products have bisoprolol as active ingredient. CHF (Congestive Heart Failure) has a specific indication for use. Bisoprolol Xpharma is a generic copy to Emconcor.

8.2 Problem to Remember

As presented elsewhere low compliance can be intentional or non-intentional. Problems to remember is typical non-intentional. Simple tools and help are summarised in Box 8.2.

Box 8.2 Tools and help patients to remember to take medications

Combine it with a daily routine like when waking up, at breakfast, to the 9 o' clock news etcetera. Food interactions must be considered (below)

Reduce the number of daily intake. Use Depot preparations or medications with longer half-life.

If appropriate use combination medications

Use calendar packages or dosing aid equipments. In some countries pharmacy pre-packed multi-dose bags (one for each scheduled time) are available.

If the patient has missed one or several doses there might be a need to overcompensate for the missing doses and to restore steady-state levels fast, but general rules are hard to give. Nowadays, this information is often available in the package leaflet for each medication. The information is also available on EMEA home page (EMEA 2008). Fore many medications there is no recommendation. For some medications like simvastatin, citalopram and atenolol the advice is not to compensate for missing doses.

If specific advice is needed and information is not available from the manufacturer information on the number of missed doses and proposed dosing schedule is needed. This information must be combined with the pharmacological properties (dynamics, kinetics, and toxicity), disease- and patient characteristics.

8.3 Problem in Handling

Many elderly have vision and co-ordination problems. This is problematic for reading and opening containers and package leaflets pour solutions, dripping eye-drops etcetera. Several aids are commercially available and sold at pharmacies.

8.4 Problem to Swallow

Dry mouth is a problem among many elderly (Chapter 5). This can be an adverse drug reaction caused by anticholinergic drugs. In this case it is even more important to follow the written instructions for use. For solid oral medications it is important to take a seating or standing position before intake. Moisture first the mouth with some water, put the medication on the back of the tongue, and drink at least half a glass of water. Historically several medications (potassium, some diuretics, NSAIDs) has caused several serious oesophageal ulcers because of errors in the intake. The problems have also been connected to the pharmaceutical preparation. After reformulation the problems have decreased. Alendronate (Fosamax) tablets still cause major problems and the written instructions should be followed in detail.

Sometimes a solid oral preparation needs to be divided or crushed. Normally this is not a problem and problems should be written on the package and in the package leaflet.

The reason for the problems is often that the characteristics of the medication are changed. Depot formulation loses its slow release properties with increased peak- and decreased through concentrations. Enteric coating is destroyed with stomach irritation from the medication or destruction of the active ingredient by the acidic content of the stomach. Also there can be problems with taste, colouring, and risk with allergies and irritation mainly for the health care personals.

Administration of medication via a gastro-oesophageal tube is sometimes problematic and depends on several factors. If a medication can be divided or crushed does not automatically means that it can be given in a tube. The inner-size and position of the tube, and the physical-, chemical- and pharmacological characteristics of the drug is important. The risk is that the flow in the tube is stopped and that the effects of the medication are increased or decreased. Sometimes the formulation can be changed; solutions are normally a suitable alternative. Some guidance for administration of various formulations is given in Box8.3 and specific problems for some common medications are given in Table 8.3.

Table 8.3 Specific problems with gastro-oesophageal tube administration for selected medications

Medication	Problem	Action
Felodipin tablet	Unsuitable for dissolving since a gel is formed that blocks the tube flow	Change drug. Another calcium channel blocker
Omeprazole	Each particle in the capsule is protected by an acid stable content that must not be crushed. The granules in the capsule can be too large for tube administration.	Change drug. Another proton-pump inhibitor with smaller granules such as Nexium or Prilosec/Losec MUPS. Special instructions are available
Sucralphate	Should not be given in a duodenal tube since the effect is directly on a damaged mucosa in the stomach and pylorus.	Change drug if the tube ends in the duodenum.

Box 8.3 Guidance for administration of various formulations in Gastro-oesophageal tubes

Use gloves, single-use syringes and mouth protection
Control the position of the tube
Use as a first alternative solutions or water soluble tablets. Avoid entero- and depot formulations, and capsules that not can be opened.
Administer as a bolus directly into the tube.
Do not administer more than one medication simultaneously.
Mix thick mixtures with equal amount of water. Crush the tablet, open and empty the capsule, dissolve with 20 ml water. NB Also the undissolved content should normally be given.
Rinse with 20 ml water before and after the tube administration.

8.5 Food Interactions

Food can interact with drugs, but drugs can also interact with food. Examples of the latter are decreased absorption and elimination of vitamins and minerals, decreased motility, and also taste-, appetite- and vomiting problems (Box 8.4).

Box 8.4 Examples of drugs that can affect food intake

Diuretics, ACE-inhibitors and NSAID affects the elimination of electrolytes

Amphetamine, ephedrine and some SSRI can reduce appetite.

Tramadol, dopaminagonists and many antibacterial can cause nausea and vomiting.

Metoclopramide, neurolepics and erythromycin increases gastro-intestinal motility; can give pain and affect absorption of nutrition's

Anticholinergics decreases gastro-intestinal motility.

Zopiclone, levodopa, metronidazole, metformin, and paroxetine, can disturb the taste.

Interaction by food on the drugs adds additional variability and un-certainties to drug absorption and there are several classical examples of serious interactions (Table 8.4).

Table 8.4 Examples of serious interactions between food and drugs

Interaction	Comment
Warfarine and green leaf vegetables	Warfarin is a K-vitamin antagonist used to decrease blood clothing and reduce risk of thrombosis. Warfarin has a narrow therapeutic interval. Food with a high K-vitamin content such as green leaf vegetables, strawberries, liver etcetera counteract the Warfarin effects.
Grapefruit juice and cyclosporine	Cyclosporine is an immunomodulating agent used mainly to inhibit rejection after transplantations and it has a narrow therapeutic interval. Grapefruit juice is a strong inhibitor of the cyclosporine metabolism (CYP 3A4) and increases the blood concentration of cyclosporine. This can lead to toxicity but can also be used to reduce the doses and decrease the costs of the cyclosporine treatment.
Non-selective MAO-inhibitors and food rich in tyramine content.	Tyramine is an amino acid which is present in large quantities in protein rich, fermented and stored products like some cheeses, sausages, red wines, beers etcetera. Tyramine is metabolized into nor-adrenaline by the enzyme mono-amino-oxidase (MAO). If MAO is inhibited by drugs nor-adrenaline is accumulated and can give hypertensive crises.

The physiological changes and other aspects in the elderly makes this even more complicated. Example of this is decreased stomach acidity; decreased motility; decreased blood-flow to liver and gastrointestinal tract; changed pharmacokinetics and –dynamics; polypharmacy; swallowing problems; bad nutritional status; and lack of documentation.

Information on the timing between drugs and food should be written on the package or on the package leaflets. The background for this information is often hard to understand and often based only on experiences from what have been performed in the clinical trial program. Nowadays the authorities demand studies with and without food and for newer drugs this information is available in the short product characteristics (SPC) on the EMEA home page (EMEA 2008).

Most patients with chronic disease states and regular medications take their drugs according to a routine that fits them; at breakfast, lunch, dinner and at night etcetera. Often this is un-problematic; the simultaneous food intake slows the absorption but the total amount absorbed drug that reaches the central body compartments is not changed. But there are exceptions as shown in Table 8.5. If a patient takes several drugs it is reasonable to take these together with food. Potential discomfort from the stomach can be minimised and the risk to forget the doses is decreased.

The drugs that have to be taken separated from food intake are pin-pointed and the patient gets clear instructions.

Table 8.5 Examples of drugs that should or should not be taken with food

Timing with food	Drug or class	Background
Fasting conditions/between meals	Sucralfat	Acid is needed to activate sucralfat; bind to the mucosa and protect it against the acid.
	Some penicillin and anti-HIV agents.	Increased absorption and bioavailability
	Bisfosfonates, quinolones and tetracyklin	Insoluble complex with ions like Ca, Fe, Zn in milk, meat, vegetables. Decreased absorption and bioavailability
With food or direct after food	Nitrofurantoin, some cephalosporines	Increased absorption and bioavailability
	Doxycyklin, some penicillins and cephalosporines, and Nitrofurantoin	Decreases gastro-intestinal problems
	Pancrease enzymes	Supposed to have effects during the food intake.
	Misoprostol, bromocriptine, metformin and valproate.	Decreased gastro-intestinal upsets.
Just before food intake	Anti-diabetic agents	Supposed to have effect during the food intake

8.6 Short Use Before Date

A drug must be marked with a manufacturing number (batch number) and a use before date (expire date) as shown in Picture 8.1. The latter in normally dependent only on the chemical stability of the active substance. Solid preparations can normally be used up to the expire date even when the container is opened. Deviation is for example nitro-glycerine preparations and this should be written on the container. Fluid preparations (mixtures, injection solutions etc.) normally have a shorter usage time after the container is opened, because of microbiological limitations. The maximum usage time after manufacturing of a drug is five years. A drug with five years usage time can therefore be expected to have a longer usage time and a couple of months longer use is not a problem. If a drug has a shorter use before time than five years this means that at least 95% of the active substance remains at the time of expiration. The shorter the usage time the more important to not pass the written expire date. The use before time in opened containers and after preparation depends on purity demands for the pharmaceutical formulation, route for administration, storage conditions (i.e. temperature, light), type of container etc.

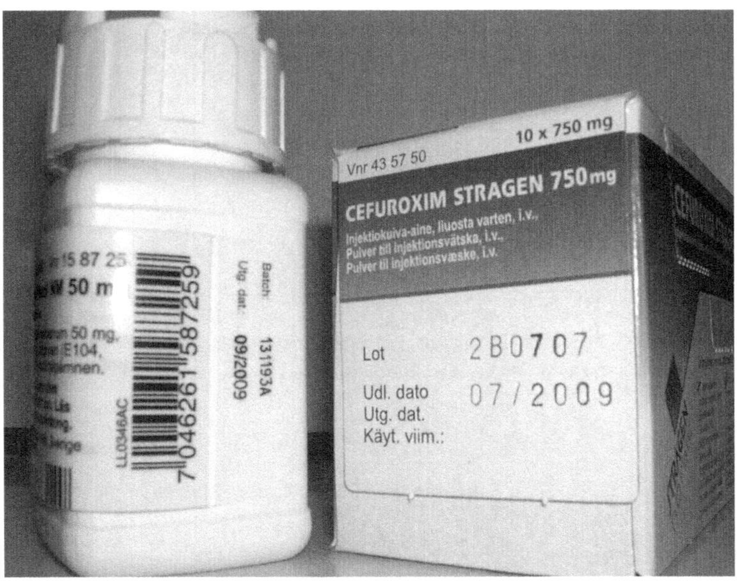

Picture 8.1 Example of containers with manufacturing number (batch number) and a use before date (expire date, in Swedish anv. före)

8.7 Conclusions

- There are many practical problems to correct drug use and intake. For the elderly this is a specific problem due to several reasons
- For good compliance and to avoid injuries these potential problems must be explored systematically and regularly for each patient
- There are several aids and methods for improvement available

References

Christians U, First MR, Benet LZ (2000) Recommendations for bioequivalence testing of cyclosporine generics revisited. Ther Drug Monit 22: 330–335

CPMP (2000) European Medicines Agency. Committee for Proprietary Medicinal Products. Note for guidance on the investigation on bioavailability and bioequivalence. CPMP/EWP/QWP/1401/98.http://www.emea.europa.eu/pdfs/human/qwp/140198en.pdf. Cited 30 Dec 2008

EU (2001) EU directive 2001/83/EC. http://eur-lex.europa.eu/LexUriServ/site/en/consleg/2001/L/02001L0083-20070126-en.pdf. Cited 30 Dec 2008

EMEA (2008) European Medicines Agency. EPARs for authorised medicinal products for human use. http://www.emea.europa.eu/htms/human/epar/a.htm. Cited 30 Dec 2008

ICH (2008) The International Conference on Harmonisation of Technical Requirements for Registration of Pharmaceuticals for Human Use (ICH). http://www.ich.org. Cited 30 Dec 2008

ISMP (2005) The Institute for Safe Medication Practices. List of confused drug names. http://www.ismp.org/Tools/confuseddrugnames.pdf. Cited 30 Dec 2008

Chapter 9
Compliance and Concordance

Abstract On average 50% of patients are compliant to long term medication treatment. Non-compliance is a drug-related problem as it may result in negative outcomes for the patient. Non-compliance can be intentional or non-intentional and related to knowledge, attitudes, and also practical problems including memory and administration difficulties. The decision to take a medication or not (compliance) lay in the hand of the patient, but the health care providers can support the patient in this decision with the aim to improve the patients' health. Definitions and tools to detect negative patient and health-care behaviour and methods for concordance are presented in this chapter.

Keywords Compliance · Concordance · Knowledge · Attitudes

9.1 Introduction

Adherence to medication is one of the most intriguing and complex behaviours demonstrated by patients (Hughes 2004). As a mean 50% of the patients are compliant to long term medication treatment (Haynes et al. 2005). Non-compliance is a drug-related problem as it may result in negative outcomes for patients. It may be compounded in populations with multiple morbidities which require multiple drug therapy. Such a population is exemplified by the elderly. It has been shown that physicians have difficulties in appraising the compliance behaviour of their patients (George et al. 1998).

Sometimes it is argued that it is a good thing that patients do not take the drugs they are prescribed. Polypharmacy, interactions and adverse drug reaction are stated to be the problem. There are at least two major arguments against this.

First; if the compliance is low the risk is that the prescriber need to increase the dose, add new drugs, or need to challenge a correct diagnosis. This cost time and money.

Second; what is happening when a patient with polypharmacy and low compliance is admitted to hospital-, or to a nursing home care? The patient gets all

P. Midlöv et al., *Drug-Related Problems in the Elderly*,
DOI 10.1007/978-90-481-2446-6_9, © Springer Science+Business Media B.V. 2009

prescribed drug with the potential of severe adverse drug reactions from over-medication.

9.2 From Compliance to Concordance

Adherence to (or compliance with) a medication regimen is generally defined as the extent to which patients take medications as prescribed by their health care providers (Osterberg and Blaschke 2005). There was a switch from the word "compliance" to "adherence" because compliance suggests that the patient is passively following the doctor's orders and that the treatment plan is not based on a therapeutic alliance or contract established between the patient and the physician. A further step was taken when the word "concordance" was first introduced in 1997 (Royal Pharmaceutical Society 1997). This was expressed as "The clinical encounter is concerned with two sets of contrasted but equally cogent health beliefs—that of the patient and that of the doctor. The task of the patient is to convey her or his health beliefs to the doctor; and of the doctor, to enable this to happen. The task of the doctor or other prescriber is to convey his or her (professionally informed) health beliefs to the patient; and of the patient, to entertain these. The intention is to assist the patient to make as informed a choice as possible about the diagnosis and treatment, about benefit and risk and to take full part in a therapeutic alliance. Although reciprocal, this is an alliance in which the most important determinations are agreed to be those that are made by the patient".

Concordance focuses on the patient-prescriber alliance and partnership. Concordance is about the patients being empowered to manage their own life and to be satisfied with a consultation. This is sometimes very difficult for the health care professionals, especially pharmacists and doctors. It means that if patients come to informed decisions that they do not want to take their medicines or that they do not want to take them in the way that research and science suggests that they should, that decision has to be accepted without dismissing or rejecting the patient. In other words, the patient may reject the medicine but the pharmacist or doctor should not reject the patient because of this decision. On the contrary, the challenge is to stay with the patient, while remaining true to what we believe about medical science. That is difficult for health care professionals and it is an enormous change from anything that has happened before. Another difficulty is that, although the word concordance is used widely now, it is occasionally used as a synonym for compliance. They are totally different words and meanings. Compliance can be seen as the objective and concordance the method as presented in Picture 9.1.

9.3 Compliance/Adherence in the Elderly

Non-adherence may not be more prevalent in older patients and there is no consensus in the literature that age is a predictor of poor adherence (Hughes 2004). Indeed, older patients may deliberately choose not to adhere to medication

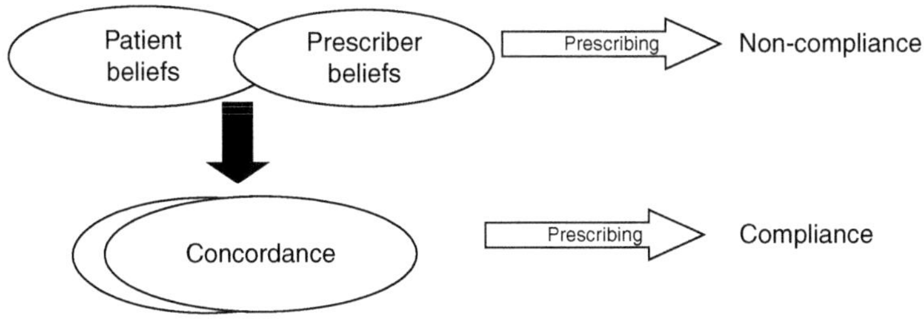

Picture 9.1 Concordance as a method for improved compliance

(intentional non-adherence) to avoid adverse effects. Furthermore, many of the studies on adherence lack commonality in terms of how adherence is measured, the definition of an "older" patient and the range of disease states which have been examined. Adherence may also be affected by access to medications which may be restricted by the use of formularies or insurance programmes. However, non-adherence may represent a greater risk in older people resulting in poor disease control which may be compounded with multiple morbidity and polypharmacy (Hughes 2004).

9.4 Clinical Consequences

There are evidences that low compliance results in hospital admissions (Williams et al. 1999, Hope et al. 2004, Sokol et al. 2005, Granger et al. 2005), mortality (Horwitz et al.1990, Osterberg and Blaschke 2005, Granger et al. 2005) and costs (Osterberg and Blaschke 2005, Sokol et al. 2005). In a study on 7599 patients with heart failure it was shown that patient compliant to candesartan (and also placebo, but to a lower extent) had a lower mortality and also lower level of admissions to hospital compared to the patients with low compliance (Granger et al. 2005). This correlation has also been shown previously (Horwitz et al.1990, CDP Research Group 1980). In a WHO report it is concluded that "improving the effect of compliance interventions can have a much larger impact on the population's health than any specific medical intervention" (WHO 2003). Good adherence to drug therapy is associated with positive health outcomes. Moreover, the observed association between good adherence to placebo and mortality supports the existence of the "healthy adherer" effect, whereby adherence to drug therapy may be a surrogate marker for overall healthy behaviour.

Based on this the concept "healthy adherer" has been introduced (Simpson et al. 2006). Recently the direct long time survival advantages of improved compliance to EBM based treatments (but not to non-EBM based) has been demonstrated in a very large study (Rasmussen et al. 2007).

9.5 Practical Problems

Problems with handling, administration, confusing names, and adverse effects can affect compliance and concordance. This has been described in Chapter 8.

9.6 Knowledge, Attitudes and Motivation

The patient knowledge, attitudes and motivation towards their treatment is often complicated. Lack of knowledge and negative attitudes (Horne and Weinman 1999, Horne et al. 1999) are important factors affecting the patient decision to take or not to take the medication according to the prescription. Positive attitudes to drug treatment have a positive correlation with compliance, and worries and concerns have a negative (Horne and Weinman 1999, Horne et al. 1999, Aikens et al. 2005). Attitudes, motivation and knowledge belong to the most important patient related factors for a good compliance (Blenkinsopp et al. 1997, WHO 2003). The most important factor for the patient in the decision to take a drug or not is believed to be the patients basic attitudes towards their medications (Blenkinsopp et al. 1997).

9.7 Tools to Detect Problems Related to Non-compliance

The patient problems related to the use of their drugs can include wrong medication, doses, dosing interval, practical problems in handling and administration, knowledge, attitudes and compliance. There are several individual tools and strategies in the literature. In this section the components included in the "Medication Interview" tool is presented because it is developed by our group and since it, to our knowledge is the only tool that combines "all" patient use aspects. The 'Medication Interview' questionnaire is structured and has been developed based on literature review, searching for validated already used questionnaires. Relevant questionnaires have been put together into a tool for identification of problems related to errors in the medication chart, in the patients practical handling of their medications at home, knowledge, attitudes (BMQ) and compliance (Morisky 4-item scale). A brief presentation is given below and a more detailed description of the tools and an evaluation of the use has been published by our group (Bondesson et al. 2009)

"Morisky four item scale" (Morisky et al. 1986) assesses the patient compliance. This validated questionnaire includes four questions. The theory underlying this measure is that non-compliance may result from forgetting, carelessness, stopping the drug when feeling better or stopping when feeling worse. According to this scale patients may be classified as low, medium or high compliant.

"The beliefs about medicines questionnaire (BMQ) –specific" (Horne and Weinman 1999, Horne et al. 1999) captures the patients attitudes towards their drug treatment. BMQ is a validated instrument made up by two parts, necessity and concerns, consisting of five assertions each. An indication of the relative importance of these attitudes for the individual patient may be obtained by calculating the necessity-concerns differential.

No validated questionnaires asking the patient direct questions about the indication for each medication were found. For each drug we therefore let the patient specify against which disease or symptom each medicine was taken. Discrepancies in the patient drug use and knowledge of each medication is revealed, comparing drug use stated by the patient by the medical charts, and by other available sources.

9.8 Interventions for Improvement

There are some external evidences from systematic research in the field. As for other Evidence based medicines principles, these evidences have to be used together with the knowledge of the individual patient characteristics. As described previously the physicians have difficulties in appraising the compliance behaviour of their patients. Therefore it is important to identify possible non-compliance based also on knowledge, attitudes and motivational aspects as described above.

There are some systematic reviews in the field as presented below and a guidance (Nice Guidance 2008) is available as of January 2009.

9.8.1 Systematic Reviews of Strategies to Improve Compliance in the Elderly

A range of strategies have been implemented to try and improve adherence in the elderly population (Hughes 2004). This includes; the use of forgiving drugs (those which have a prescribed dosage interval that is 50% or less the duration of drug action); drug holidays; once-daily scheduling, supplemented through the use of compliance aids; therapeutic alliance between the patient and healthcare professional (concordance), multifaceted interventions including practical approaches.

A range of behavioural, educational and provider-focused strategies have also been tested, individually or in combination, for improving medication adherence. This has been analysed in several systematic reviews. In a very recent (Elliott et al. 2008) it was stated that Pharmaceutical care was the model for the interventions used in the majority of the studies. Only four out of eight included studies demonstrated a significant improvement in adherence as a result of the interventions. Regular scheduled patient follow-up along with a multi-compartment dose administration aid was an effective strategy for maintaining adherence in one study, while group education combined with individualised medication cards was successful in another study. Medication review by pharmacists with a focus on regimen simplification was found to be effective in two studies. The researchers were unable to draw firm conclusions in favour of any particular intervention and they concluded that innovative strategies for enhancing medication adherence in the elderly and reliable measures of adherence are needed. Until further evidence from single-intervention strategies becomes available they recommend combinations of educational and behavioural strategies.

9.8.2 Communicating Evidences for Benefit and Harm

Informed patients are more likely to actively participate in their care, make wiser decisions, come to a common understanding with their physicians, and adhere more fully to treatment as described above. According to a systematic review (Epstein et al. 2004) there is a paucity of evidence to guide how physicians can most effectively share clinical evidence with patients facing decisions. They recommend accomplishing five communication tasks to address in framing and communicating clinical evidence: understanding the patient's (and family members') experience and expectations; building partnership; providing evidence, including a balanced discussion of uncertainties; presenting recommendations informed by clinical judgment and patient preferences; and checking for understanding and agreement. The review also concluded that relative risk reductions as a source for information may be misleading; absolute risk is preferred (see Chapter 3). Less-educated and older patients preferred proportions to percentages and did not appreciate confidence intervals

9.8.3 Motivational Interviewing

Positive effects of "Motivational Interviewing" have been shown in small studies (Possidente et al. 2005). It is designed for assisting patients to commit to change, based on a patient's motivation and readiness to alter behaviour. The "motivational" part of the term underscores the fact that motivation is fundamental to change. An individual must be ready, willing, and able to change. The word "interviewing" differentiates this method from treatment or counselling and enables patients and providers to examine events together. It is described like two people sitting side by side, paging through an album of family pictures. The storyteller turns the page; the listener wants to learn and understand and, as such, may ask questions. Systematic practice models and studies are needed to further explore the benefits and cost-effectiveness.

9.9 Conclusions

- Only 50% of patients are compliant to long term medication treatment
- Non-compliance is a drug-related problem as it may result in negative outcomes for the patient. This has been proven in very large studies
- Attitudes, motivation and knowledge belong to the most important patient related factors for a good compliance and patient-prescriber alliance and

partnership (concordance) is very important as a base for patient-empowerment and responsibility

- Non-adherence may represent a greater risk in the elderly and there are often practical problems
- Interventions for improved compliance interventions can have a much larger impact on the population's health than any specific medical intervention

References

Aikens JE, Nease Jr DE et al. (2005) Adherence to maintenance-phase antidepressant medication as a function of patient beliefs about medication. Ann Fam Med 3: 23–30

Blenkinsopp A, Bond C, Britten N (1997) From compliance to concordance. Achieving shared goals in medicine taking. Royal Pharmaceutical Society of Great Britain and Merck Sharpe & Dome, London UK

Bondesson Å, Hellström L, Eriksson T, Höglund P (2009) A structured questionnaire to asses patient compliance and beliefs about medicines taken account of the ordered categorical structure of data. J Eval Clin Pract (in press)

CDP (1980) Coronary Drug Project Research Group. Influence of adherence to treatment and response of cholesterol on mortality in the coronary drug project. N Engl J Med 303: 1038–1041

Elliott RA and Stewart DC (2008) A systematic review of interventions to improve medication taking in elderly patients prescribed multiple medications. Drugs Aging 25: 307–324

Epstein RM, Alper BS, Quill TE (2004) Communicating evidence for participatory decision making. JAMA 291: 2359–2366

George J, Goldberg AI, Cohen G, Rubin AH (1998) Physician assessments of patient compliance with medical treatment. Soc Sci Med 47: 1873–1876

Granger BB, Swedberg K, Ekman I, Granger CB, Olofsson B et al. (2005) Adherence to candesartan and placebo and outcomes in chronic heart failure in the CHARM program: double-blind, randomised, controlled clinical trial. Lancet 366: 2005–2011

Haynes RB, Yao X, Degani A, Kripalani S, Garg A, McDonald HP (2005) Interventions to enhance medication adherence. Cochrane Database Syst Rev 19 (4): CD000011

Hope CJ, Wu J, Tu W et al. (2004) Association of medication adherence, knowledge, and skills with emergency department visits by adults 50 years or older with congestive heart failure. Am J Health Syst Pharm 61: 2043–2049

Horne R and Weinman J (1999) Patients beliefs about prescribed medicines and their role in adherence to treatment in chronic physical illness. J Psychosom Res 47: 555–567

Horne R, Weinman J, Hankins M (1999) The beliefs about medicines questionnaire: The development and evaluation of a new method for assessing the cognitive representation of medication. Psychol and Health 14: 1–24

Horwitz RI, Viscoli CM, Berkman L et al. (1990) Treatment adherence and risk of death after a myocardial infarction. Lancet 336: 542–545

Hughes CM (2004) Medication non-adherence in the elderly: how big is the problem? Drugs Aging 21: 793–811

Morisky DE, Green LW, Levine DM (1986) Concurrent and predictive validity of a self-reported measure of medication adherence. Med Care 24: 67–74

NICE Guidance (2008) National Institute for Health and Clinical Excellence. Guidance Medicines concordance. http://www.nice.org.uk/guidance/index.jsp?action=byID&o=11638. Cited 30 Dec 2008

Osterberg L and Blaschke T (2005) Adherence to medication. N Engl J Med 353: 487–497

Possidente CJ, Bucci KK, McClain WJ (2005) Motivational interviewing: a tool to improve medication adherence? Am J Health Syst Pharm 62: 1311–1314

Royal Pharmaceutical Society (1997) From compliance to concordance: towards shared goals in medicine taking. Royal Pharmaceutical Society of Great Britain, London

Rasmussen JN, Chong A, Alter DA (2007) Relationship between adherence to evidence-based pharmacotherapy and long-term mortality after acute myocardial infarction. JAMA 297: 177–186

Simpson SH, Eurich DT, Majumdar SR, Padwal RS, Tsuyuki RT, Varney J, Johnson JA (2006) A meta-analysis of the association between adherence to drug therapy and mortality. BMJ 33: 15–20

Sokol MC, McGuigan KA, Verbrugge RR, Epstein RS (2005) Impact of medication adherence on hospitalization risk and healthcare cost. Med Care 43: 521–530

WHO (2003) Adherence to long-term therapies: evidence for action. World Health Organisation, WHO Press, New York

Williams BR, Nichol MB, Lowe B, Yoon PS, McCombs JS, Margolies J (1999) Medication use in residential care facilities for the elderly. Ann Pharmacother 33: 149–155

Chapter 10
Strategies and Interventions for Improvement

Abstract For the elderly the health-related quality of life is often reduced. Since health status often is related to medication use (symptom control vs. adverse drug effects and other problems related to medications) a process without uncontrolled hazardous and important errors is crucial. Problems and some methods to accomplish this have been presented in this book. In this chapter we focus on general strategies for research and development, and also approaches and processes for delivery of care, important for medication use in the elderly. This includes information technology support, evidence based sources and practical tools and models for identification, resolving and prevention of a patients drug-related problems. The tools and models include "pharmaceutical care and medicines management", "medication reconciliation", "medication review" and "trigger tools". We also present some aspects of the future possibilities including personalised medicine.

Keywords Pharmaceutical care · Medicines management · Medication reconciliation · Medication review · Information technology · Personalised medicine · Trigger tools

10.1 Introduction

Research and development of delivery of care is complicated and the interventions normally need to be multi professional and team based, targeted towards large groups of professionals and complex also in other aspects. Medical Research Council in Great Britain has published a report for development and evaluation of complex intervention that can be of great help (MRC 2008). A control group and especially randomisation is problematic when researching a team approach. Another problem is funding for larger studies with appropriate outcome and power. As presented in Chapter 3, the quality of care from structure, to process and outcome is also fundamental to research (Donobedian 2003).

Below we have listed some very important aspects for improving quality of care in the elderly. We also list or explain some models or practical approaches for improvement.

P. Midlöv et al., *Drug-Related Problems in the Elderly*,
DOI 10.1007/978-90-481-2446-6_10,

10.2 Information Technology Development Within Health Care

Imagine a fully developed IT system where all important information on an individual person's health-related aspects are stored, easy searchable and safely available for communication and systematic support for decisions and also follow up of interventions, by the patient and health care providers. Of course there are several potential drawbacks to this but from a patient health care perspective the benefits are clear. In UK a large scale IT project "Connecting for Health" are supposed to support the UK-NHS in providing better, safer care, by delivering computer systems and services that improve how patient information is stored and accessed (NHS 2004). This could be one way to start up. However the patient perspective on, communication, learning, responsibility, knowledge, follow-up on effects etcetera must be supported.

It is important to state that information technology does not solve all problems connected to communicating and documenting problems in the use and handling of drugs. It has been stated that electronic communication between the general practitioner (GP) and the community pharmacists improve agreement but does not suffice as a solution to obtain reliable information (van der Kam et al. 2001). Also GPs found discharge content more important than delivery method (Pillai et al. 2004). Therefore we need to build the improvements of the patient needs and use IT as a tool for further improvement of overall safety and quality as described previously.

10.3 Evidence Based Database Sources for Effective Clinical Practices

There are several international and national databases freely available. Most guidance is on the selection of appropriate medications on external evidences (See EBM in Chapter 3). Cochrane Reviews is an international database including EBM evaluation on clinical practices, and NICE is a national source with high impact on practice even outside England/Wales. In some countries databases on national guidance are provided.

10.3.1 Cochrane

In the Cochrane Reviews database 81 protocols and reviews are available (Cochrane Reviews database). This includes continuing education and quality assurance (16 documents), financial interventions (7), organisational interventions (26), and reviews of interventions to improve specific types of practices (28). Several of the documents involve practices with elderly and medications focus. Specific focus can be found in four of the protocols

- Care home versus hospital and own homes environment for rehabilitation older people

- Effectiveness of shared care across the interface between primary and speciality care in chronic disease management
- Discharge planning
- Expanding the role of outpatient pharmacists: effects on health services utilisation, costs, and patient outcomes

10.3.2 NICE

National Institute for Health and Clinical Excellence (NICE) produces guidance on public health, health technologies and clinical practice, including various clinical and optimal practice topics (Nice Guidance 2007). They provide recommendations for the treatment and care of people by health professionals, to develop standards to assess the clinical practice of individual health professionals, in the education and training of health professionals, to help patients make informed decisions improve communication between patient and health professional etcetera. For each topic, help and tools for implementing guidance is provided such as cost templates, audit criteria and slide sets. This also includes implementation tools, commissioning guides—supporting clinical service redesign, and optimal practice review: recommendation reminders.

Examples of guidance on medication and elderly are Medication reconciliation, and also Medication concordance.

10.4 Pharmaceutical Care and Medicines Management

Pharmaceutical care (PC) is defined by Hepler and Strand (1990) as "the responsible provision of drug therapy for the purpose of achieving definite outcomes that improve a patient's quality of life". PC involves three major functions on behalf of the patient:

- Identifying potential and actual drug-related problems
- Resolving actual drug-related problems
- Preventing potential drug-related problems

Like Medical Care, Nursing Care etcetera PC consists of core components; the philosophy, the patient care process, and the practical management system to support the practice. PC was developed from Clinical Pharmacy Services (see below) with more focus on the patients need and on the practitioners (pharmacist) responsibilities towards the patient and the outcome of the drug therapy. To be able to show the improved process of care a categorisation system for drug-related problems was developed. The taxonomy has been further developed into seven categories (Cipolle et al. 1998). This can be used for practice and in studies.

- Need for additional drug therapy
- Unnecessary drug therapy

- Wrong drug
- Dosage too low
- Adverse drug reaction
- Dose too high
- Compliance

PC can be a team approach but can also be practiced by individuals. Pharmacists are the profession which has adopted PC as their responsibility and most studies has been on effects on various clinical pharmacy practice models. The possible interventions in PC are unlimited.

Medicines Management (MM) is a terminology used for Pharmaceutical Care (PC) in the United Kingdom (except Scotland). The background and differences have been described (Simpson 2001). PC is MM, but MM is not necessarily PC. The department of MM at Keele University has adopted the definition "Medicines Management seeks to maximise health gain through the optimum use of medicines. It encompasses all aspects of medicines use, from the prescribing of medicines through the ways in which medicines are taken or not taken by patients".

The development of community pharmacy in England, according to the National Health Service is focused on MM. The service includes Medication Review, support for patients with particular medication needs, and structured MM services. The latter includes a structured assessment of the patient's prescribed medicines with a view to discussing the matter with the patient's general practitioner. The topics for discussion with the GP may include such matters as drug interactions, side effects, polypharmacy and whether a more effective drug regimen could be implemented. Discussions between the patient and the pharmacist will take place at regular intervals for the purpose of reviewing treatment. Patients will be advised on how to use their medicines and other steps they can take to cope with their condition.

Integrated Medicines Management (IMM) is seamless PC (Scullin et al. 2007). It includes Medicines Management (Clinical Pharmacy Services) but also exchange of information over the primary/secondary care interface, Medication Reconciliation, and patient education for improved adherence. The IMM model has been tested in Northern Ireland and has been shown to be very effective in reducing length of hospital stay, decrease rate of re-admission. NNT for readmission over one year was calculated at 12. The model is now under investigation in Sweden, and improved medication appropriateness has been shown (Bergkvist et al. 2009).

10.5 Medication Reconciliation

Medication Reconciliation is defined as "The process of identifying the most accurate list of a patient's current medicines- including the name, dosage, frequency, and route- and comparing them to the current list in use, recognizing any discrepancies, and documenting any changes thus resulting in a complete list of medications, accurately communicated" (IHI MedReconcilliation 2008). Establishing these details may involve discussion with the patient and/or carers and the use of records from primary care or from pharmacy. Different sources for information are available in different countries, regions or counties. Medication Reconciliation does not include Medication Review.

Patients, in particular the elderly, are moved between different settings in the health care system. Medicines are involved in most of the stages of the journey. This includes: home to hospital, home to care home or hospice, home to day centre, hospital to home, hospital to care home or hospice, ward to ward in hospital, hospital to hospital, care home to home, care home to care home. Especially on admission to, and discharge from, hospital there are several factors that can lead to errors.

Experience from hundreds of organisations has shown that poor communication of medical information at transition points is responsible for as many as 50% of all medication errors in the hospital and up to 20% of adverse drug events (IHI MedReconcilliation 2008). In our different settings at a university and county hospitals, we had errors in 40–85% of the elderly patients before starting a new practice.

Each time a patient moves from one setting to another, clinicians should compare previous medication orders with new orders and plans for care and reconcile any differences. If this process does not occur in a standardised manner designed to ensure complete reconciliation, medication errors may lead to adverse events and harm (IHI MedReconcilliation 2008). Several national organisations round the world have now produced help to reduce errors with medication reconciliation. Some examples are given below.

- IHI has produced a full package for improvement with tool kits, follow up measures on all aspects on Medication Reconciliation. Based on different strategies and settings they also report an error rate reduction of at least 50% (IHI MedReconcilliation 2008)
- NICE has produced an evidence based background and technical patient solutions for Medicines Reconciliation on admission to hospital (NICE 2007). In addition to specifying standardised systems for collecting and documenting information about current medications, policies for medicines reconciliation on admission they state that it should be ensure that:
  - pharmacists are involved in medicines reconciliation as soon as possible after admission
  - the responsibilities of pharmacists and other staff in the Medicines Reconciliation process are clearly defined; these responsibilities may differ between clinical areas
  - strategies are incorporated to obtain information about medications for people with communication difficulties
- We have produced a tool “Medication Report in Discharge Information for patients” that reduced error rates and health-care contacts based on these errors by 50% in elderly patients (Midlöv et al. 2008a,b).

10.6 Medication Review

There is no single agreed definition of Medication Review. According to National Health Services in UK it is "A structured critical examination of the patient's medicines with the objective of reaching agreement with the patient about treatment, optimising the impact of medicines, minimising the number of medication-related problems and reducing waste" (NHS 2005). The review is undertaken in a systematic way by a competent person, documented and monitored. It can be conducted in the patient's home, in a hospital ward, in a pharmacy etc. and it can be included in pharmaceutical benefit systems as a base for accreditation and reimbursement. Medication review is the base for Pharmaceutical Care and the process has been described in detail (Cipolle et al. 1998). Several studies and reviews have shown the benefit of Medication Reviews as part of clinical pharmacy programs (Bond et al. 2001, Schumock et al. 1996, 2003, Morrison and Wertheimer 2001, Scullin et al. 2007). However there are also studies showing negative results for example home based reviews performed by community pharmacists (Holland et al. 2005). This puts focus on the importance of a powerful intervention, training of the involved, access to correct information, and the probable need for a team approach.

10.7 Trigger Tools

Detecting the incidence and type of adverse drug events (ADEs) and medication errors is important for improving the quality of health care delivery. Problems include missing dose, wrong dose, frequency, and route errors. The consequence (ADE) of the errors depends on medication and patient factors as described previously. Some of these problems are organisational and related to chart order system and prescribing.

ADEs and medication errors can be extracted from practice data, incidents reports from health professionals, and patient surveys. Practice data include charts, laboratory, prescription data, and administrative databases, and can be reviewed manually or screened by computer systems to identify signals. A method of ADE and medication error detection and classification has been presented that is feasible and has good reliability (Marimoto et al. 2004). It can be used in various clinical settings to measure and improve medication safety.

The use of "triggers," or clues, to identify adverse drug events (ADEs) is an effective method for measuring the overall level of harm from medications in a health care organisation. Trigger tools are an easy-to-use method for accurately identifying ADEs—harm from medications—and measuring the rate of ADEs over time (IHI Trigger Tools 2008). Measuring ADE over time is a useful way to tell if changes a team is making are improving the safety of the medication system and is used by hundreds of hospitals especially in the USA. It measures the level of harm from each ADE, and identifies areas for improvement in the organisations. Also interactive

Trigger Tools are available. A list of shared trigger tools for use in various settings is available (IHI Trigger Tools 2008).

10.8 Personalised Medicine

Traditional medicine has been described previously and focuses on the individual patient's clinical signs and symptoms, medical and family history, and data from laboratory and imaging evaluation to diagnose and treat illnesses. Recent advances in medical- and human genetics give us more detailed understanding of the impact of genetics in disease. Large projects, for example, the Human genome project (2008) is important for understanding of the roles of genes in normal human development and physiology and has revealed single nucleotide polymorphisms (SNPs) that account for some of the genetic variability between individuals. This is the foundation for examination of genetic variation and risk for common diseases.

Personalised medicine is the concept that information about a patient's genotype or gene expression profile could be used to tailor medical care to an individual's needs. As described previously disease state and pharmacological effects of drugs can have genetic as well as environmental aspects, i.e. the patients own genotype and phenotype. The associations between structure and function, the correlations between genotype and phenotype, and the interactions among gene, drug, and environment is very interesting and can probably be of great help to improve drug therapy and to avoid drug-related problems when available. Already now, genetic typing is possible for a low cost and can be of great value for individualisation of dosing in the elderly. Example of this can be genotyping for SNPs in genes involved in the action and metabolism of warfarin, genetic variants in the gene encoding Cytochrome P450 enzyme for important medications such as antidepressants and antipsychotics. Yan has provided a review in this area (Yan 2008). For an up-date of evidences in the area he also recommends an integrated search engine which also includes a collections of tools (Pharm Tao 2008).

10.9 Conclusions

- Improving quality of medication care in the elderly requires systematic processes for the team responsible for the patient care and also for individualisation of each patients care
- Evidence based tools and models should be the base if possible
- The patient individualisation should include activities for identification, resolving and preventing drug-related problems as described by pharmaceutical care and medication review and possible with the additional personalised medicine support
- The professional and team approach should be targeted in the same direction and appropriate systematic approaches such as trigger tools, medication- reconciliation and review should be used

- The health care system also need to build an IT system supportive to the processes and tools used

References

Bergkvist A, Midlöv P, Höglund P, Larsson L, Eriksson T (2009) A multi-intervention approach on drug therapy can lead to more appropriate drug use in the elderly. J Eval Clin Pract (in press)
Bond CA, Raehl CL, Franke T (2001) Intercorrelationship among mortality rates, drug costs, total costs of care, and length of stay in US hospitals. Pharmacotherapy 21: 129–141
Cipolle RJ, Strand LM, Moreley PC (1998) Pharmaceutical care practice. McGraw-Hill, New York
Cochrane Reviews (2008) Database. Effective. Practices and Organisations of Care. http://www.mrw.interscience.wiley.com/cochrane/cochrane_clsysrev_subjects_fs.html. Cited 30 Dec 2008
Donobedian A (2003) An introduction to quality assurance in health care. Oxford University Press, New York
Hepler CD and Strand LM (1990) Opportunities and responsibilities in pharmaceutical care. Am J Hosp Pharm 47: 533–543
Holland R, Lenaghan E, Harvey I, Smith R, Shepstone L, Lipp A, Christou M, Evans D, Hand C (2005) Does home based medication review keep older people out of hospital? The HOMER randomised controlled trial. BMJ 330: 293–298
Human Genome Project (2008)http://www.ornl.gov/sci/techresources/Human_Genome/home.shtml. Cited 30 Dec 2008
IHI Trigger Tools (2008) Institute for Health care Improvement. Trigger Tools for Measuring ADE. http://www.ihi.org/ihi/workspace/tools/trigger/. Cited 30 Dec 2008
IHI MedReconcilliation (2008) Institute for Health care Improvement. Prevent adverse drug events (Medication reconciliation). http://www.ihi.org/IHI/Programs/Campaign/ADEsMedReconciliation.htm. Cited 30 Dec 2008
Midlöv P, Holmdahl L, Eriksson T et al. (2008) Medication report reduces number of medication errors when elderly patients are discharged from hospital. Pharm World Sci. 30(1): 92–8
Midlöv P, Deierborg E, Holmdahl L et al. (2008) Clinical outcomes from the use of Medication Report when elderly patients are discharged from hospital. Pharm World Sci. 30(6): 840–5
Morrison A and Wertheimer AI (2001) Evaluation of studies investigating the effectiveness of pharmacists' clinical services. Am J Health-Syst Pharm 58: 569–577
MRC (2008) Medical Research Council in Great Britain. Developing and evaluating complex interventions-Guidance. http://www.mrc.ac.uk/Utilities/Documentrecord/index.htm?d=MRC004871. Cited 30 Dec 2008
NICE Guidance (2007) National Institute for Health and Clinical Excellence. Guidance. Technical patient safety solutions for medicines reconciliation on admission of adults to hospital. http://www.nice.org.uk/guidance/index.jsp?action=byID&o=11897. Cited 30 Dec 2008
NHS (2004) Connecting for Health. Connecting for health business plan: London Department of Health. http://www.connectingforhealth.nhs.uk. Cited 30 Dec 2008
NHS (2005) NHS Community Pharmacy Contractual Framework. Enhanced Service-Medication Review (Full Clinical Review). EN7, Version 1.http://www.psnc.org.uk/data/files/PharmacyContract/enhanced_service_spec/en7__medication_review.doc. Cited 30 Dec 2008
Pharm Tao (2008) The Center of Personalized and Systems Medicine. http://sysmed.pharmtao.com. Cited 30 Dec 2008
Pillai A, Thomas SS, Garg M (2004) The electronic immediate discharge document: experience from the South West of Scotland. Inform Prim Care 12: 67–73
Schumock GT, Meek PD, Ploetz PA, Vermeulen LC (1996) Economic evaluation of Clinical Pharmacy service – 1988–1995. Pharmacotherapy16: 1188–1208
Schumock GT, Butler MG, Meek PD, Ploetz PA, Vermeulen LC, Arondekar BW et al. (2003) Evidence of the economic benefit of clinical pharmacy service: 1996–2000. Pharmacotherapy 23: 113–132

Scullin C, Scott MG, Hogg A, McElnay JC (2007) An innovative approach to integrated medicines management. J Eval Clin Pract 13: 781–788

Simpson D (2001) What is medicines management and what is pharmaceutical care? Pharm J 266: 150

Van der Kam WJ, Meyboom de Jong B, Tromp TF, Moorman PW, van der Lei J (2001) Effects of electronic communication between the GP and the pharmacist. The quality of medication data on admission and after discharge. Fam Pract 18: 605–609

Yan Q (2008) The integration of personalized and systems medicine: bioinformatics support for pharmacogenomics and drug discovery. Methods Mol Biol 448: 1–19

Chapter 11
Summary and Perspectives

Abstract The health care system can help elderly people to stay healthy or to improve health if a systematic process to patient care can be provided. The first step is to look upon all new medication treatment as an experiment, and therefore continuously follow-up on the patient objectives of the treatment, documenting treatment goals and results, and communicating this with the patient and all involved health care-professionals.

In this book we have provided background for problems and examples of solutions to improve quality of medication care in the elderly. In this chapter we provide visions and objectives for further improvement in care of the elderly. We also summarise some very important practical aspects in the care of the elderly and give references to other chapters in this book.

Keywords Vision · Objective · Patient centred care

11.1 Vision and Objectives for Medication Use in the Elderly

There is no scientifically valid evidence that anti aging drugs presently on the market can increase longevity (Turnheim 2004), hence aging is still an inevitable process.

For the individual elderly the background for medication use is normally sustained or improved health. Also, based on economic constrains for the individual and for the society, a health economy perspective must be added. So the general vision for medication use could be "safe and cost-effective use for improved or sustained health". To achieve this, research and development must focus on methods aiming at more patient individualisation, and also support to patient and health care providers in a systematic way. Some objectives for the development of structures and processes could be as described in Box 11.1.

DOI 10.1007/978-90-481-2446-6_11,

Box 11.1 Some objectives for the development of structures and processes in the medication care of the elderly

1. Conscious, evidence-based and outcome oriented prescribing in concordance with the patient expectation and need to improve the patient health and quality of life
2. Let the people/patients take responsibility for their present and future health. Organise the health-care system to support this
3. Use the skills of the team and of all the professionals involved in patient care and decisions
4. Look upon all new medication treatment as an experiment, and therefore continuously follow-up on the patient objectives of the treatment, documenting treatment goals and results, and communicating this with the patient and all involved health care-professionals
5. Develop information technology (IT) systems to support the patient (responsibilities and demand), and also the health care process for better follow up on treatment in the individual patient and populations

11.2 Quality Improvement

All the objectives presented in Box 11.1 can be described as quality improvement in the structure and process to support improvement in each patient's health outcome. This support the patient medication care process presented in Fig. 3.1. Various problems and tools and models for improvement have been described in this book. Another approach to prevent medication errors and to improve care is to be open and continuously learn from mistakes. The basis for this is not to punish health care providers who make errors, as this may lead to less reporting of errors. In Britain, the government has taken steps away from this "blame-culture" (Wise 2001). In a declaration it is stated that honest failure should not be responded to primarily by blame and retribution, but by learning and by a drive to reduce risk for future patients.

11.3 Product- or Patient- Centred Treatment

The pharmaceutical industries, universities, various institutes etcetera invest hundreds of billions every year for research and development of new drugs or drug candidates. The investment for researching improvement of the actual use of drugs in the society and in individual patients is very limited compared to this. It is important to stress that a new treatment, even if more effective, not automatically improves health, especially not in the elderly population and when the practical use and handling, including compliance, is problematic. Instead of focusing on new and exciting treatment options we should maybe instead focus on the present treatment options and to improve the structure and process as described by Donobedian (Donobedian 2003).

Prevention of disease is of course very important and the individual have a responsibility for their own health in a short and long perspective. The health care system has to support the individual to make correct decision and also to further help them when disease is evident. The cornerstone to this is surgery and medication treatment. As described in Chapter 3 there are requirements for documentation of new medications when used in the elderly. However those controlled trials will always be artificial and we need more evidences and comparisons from normal clinical use based on populations and individuals. This information could be gathered continuously if the patient care supportive IT system really was supportive.

11.4 Summary of Simple Practice Conclusions

In all previous chapters we have made some conclusions. In Table 11.1 we summarise the most important potential drug-related problems to consider in each patient consultation. First consider the background for the symptom or problem. Is it caused by the medication? If treatment is needed first consider if a drug is necessary. Pharmacotherapy of the elderly is more complicated than in younger adults. It is important to state that drugs can not replace human contacts. Instead, a drug may have inhibited human contacts. We can never treat a shortage of staff in the elderly care with drugs.

Table 11.1 Summary of the most important actions to consider in each patient consultation, and reference to help in this book

Potential drug-related problems to consider	Help in this book (chapter)
Is the symptom or problem related to an adverse drug reaction?	Adverse drug reactions (2, 7)
Correct picture of all the patients' medications? Herbals and OTC?	Medication reconciliation (10), tools for intervention (9)
Is there a need for additional drug therapy?	EBM (3), common conditions (5), neuro-psychiatric disorders (6)
Is there any unnecessary drug therapy? Other options? Human contacts?	EBM (3) Inappropriate drugs (4) Delirium and dementia (6)
Is the drug selection correct? Appropriate to elderly? EBM in the elderly? Cost-benefit? Is the dosage correct? Reduced hepatic/renal function? Food- or drug- drug interactions?	EBM (3), inappropriate drugs (4), correct dose (2), food interactions (8), personalised medicine (10), renal elimination (2), common conditions (5), neuro-psychiatric disorders (6)
Compliance? Practical problems? Knowledge, attitudes?	Compliance incl. tools for intervention (9), practical problems (8)

Table 11.1 (continued)

Potential drug-related problems to consider	Help in this book (chapter)
Need for further communication, coaching and empowerment for sustained improvement of compliance?	Compliance incl. communication(9), medication reconciliation (10), calculating benefits and risks (3)
Documentation and follow up on effects!	Medication reconciliation (10), Pharmaceutical care and Medication review (10)
Communication with other professionals involved!	Medication reconciliation (10)
Communication with relatives, next of kin etcetera!	Medication reconciliation (10)

If all health care professionals always consider these potential drug-related problems the elderly will benefit more from their pharmacotherapy.

References

Donobedian A (2003) An introduction to quality assurance in health care. Oxford University Press, New York

Turnheim K (2004) Drug therapy in the elderly. Exp Gerontol 39: 1731–1738

Wise J (2001) UK government and doctors agree to end “blame culture”. BMJ 323: 9

Index

A

Absorption, 10, 11, 49, 50, 56, 66, 69, 107, 108
ACE-inhibitors, 16, 62, 63, 71, 74, 86, 107
Acetylcholine, 43
Adherence, 2, 4, 28, 111–113, 115, 122
Adverse drug event, 6, 91, 92, 94, 95, 123, 124
Adverse drug reactions, 2–4, 9, 13–17, 37, 39, 41–44, 62, 79, 91–99, 105, 111, 112, 122, 131
Adverse drug withdrawal event (ADWE), 3, 4, 17
Adverse effects, 2–4, 10, 15–17, 30, 37, 38, 40, 41, 44, 56, 83–87, 96, 113, 114
Alzheimer's disease, 24, 42, 84–87
Analogue drug, 101, 103
Anticholinergic drugs, 16, 37, 43, 50, 59–61, 81, 86, 105
Anticholinergic effects, 37–44, 53, 59, 60, 74, 81, 85, 87
Anticholinergics, 107
Antipsychotic drugs, 3, 15, 34, 37, 38, 41–44, 79, 82, 83, 87
Anxiety, 38, 40, 69, 71, 79, 83, 86
Attitudes, 111, 114–116, 131

B

Baroreceptor reflex response, 14
Beer's criteria, 37, 38, 107
Benefits, 4–6, 21–23, 27–29, 32, 33, 41, 63, 66, 98, 102, 112, 116, 120, 124, 131, 132
Benign paroxysmal positional vertigo, 73
Benzodiazepines, 3, 11, 17, 34, 37–42, 44, 65, 70, 74, 75, 79, 81–83, 85–87
Bioavailability, 10, 102, 108
Bioequivalence, 102, 103
Blood-brain barrier, 15
Body fat, 11

C

Capacity limited drugs, 12
Cholinesterase inhibitors, 61, 80, 84
Clinical pharmacy, 95, 121, 122, 124
Common conditions, 53, 56, 73, 76, 80, 131
Communication, 1, 5, 6, 12, 21, 29, 31, 33, 38, 91–93, 116, 120, 123, 132
Compliance, 4, 6, 69, 93, 98, 104, 110, 111–117, 122, 130–132
Concordance, 23, 93, 111–117, 121, 130
Constipation, 32, 43, 44, 49–51, 56, 57, 60, 75
Cost-effectiveness, 31, 32
Cystatin C, 13

D

Delirium, 15–17, 37, 39, 41, 43, 44, 56, 79–87, 131
Dementia, 2, 16, 41, 42, 71, 74, 79–81, 83–87, 131
Depot, 104–196
Depression, 43, 65, 69, 79, 83–85
Discontinuation, 17, 41, 42
Distribution, 10–12, 39
Documentation, 1, 5, 6, 24, 29–31, 33, 41, 91, 93, 102, 103, 108, 131, 132
Drug-disease interactions, 16, 33
Drug-drug interactions, 1, 3, 9, 15, 16, 24, 131
Drug monitoring, 6
Drug-related problems, 1–6, 9, 13, 91, 92, 94–96, 99, 111, 116, 119, 121, 125, 131, 132
Dry mouth, 43, 44, 50, 53, 75, 105

E

Efficacy, 1, 3, 6, 21, 23–25, 30, 41, 84, 85, 91, 92
Elimination, 9, 11–14, 16, 63, 107, 131
Epidemiology, 1, 2
Ethics, 31, 32

Evidence based medicine (EBM), 3, 4, 6, 21–29, 32, 33, 113, 115, 120, 131
Extrapyramidal side effects, 87

F
Fall prevention, 66
Falls, 14, 40, 41, 44, 49, 64–67, 74, 75, 85
Fat-free mass, 10, 11
Flow-limited drugs, 12
Fludrocortisone, 72, 73
Follow-up, 5, 29, 31, 33, 91, 93, 115, 120, 123, 129, 130, 132
Food interactions, 101, 104, 107, 131
Fractures, 40, 49, 56, 64, 65, 67–69, 75, 80
FRAX®, 68

G
Gastric ulcers, 42, 53, 54
Gastritis, 49, 53–56, 58
Gastro-oesophageal tube, 106
Generic drug, 101, 102
Genotype, 125
Glomerular filtration, 11, 13, 42, 63, 64, 75

H
Heartburn, 56
Helicobacter pylori, 53
Hiatus hernia, 53, 56–58
Homeostatic mechanism, 9, 14, 17

I
Inappropriate drugs, 33, 34, 37–44, 81, 131
Information technology (IT), 119, 120, 126, 130, 131
Insomnia, 38, 40, 41, 74

K
Knowledge, 1, 3, 4, 6, 10, 15, 17, 22, 24, 29, 34, 38, 66, 82, 83, 93, 111, 114–116, 120, 131

L
Laxatives, 50, 51, 62
Life expectancy, 2
Lithium, 11, 13, 15, 86

M
Malnutrition, 12, 69, 81, 82
Medication Appropriateness Index (MAI), 38
Medication beliefs, 4
Medication errors, 6, 17, 33, 91–93, 123, 124, 130
Medication intake, 101–110
Medication reconciliation, 6, 33, 93, 94, 119, 121–123, 125, 131, 132
Medication review, 4, 6, 115, 119, 122–124, 132
Medicines management, 119, 121, 122
Memantine, 84
Metabolism, 11, 12, 24, 39, 107, 125
Motility, 50, 51, 107, 108
Municipality care process, 5
Muscle atrophy, 70

N
Neuro-psychiatric disorders, 79–87, 131
Non-steroidal anti-inflammatory drugs (NSAIDs), 14, 16, 37, 38, 42, 44, 52–55, 57, 61–63, 72, 73, 81, 105, 107

O
Orthostatic hypotension, 49, 65, 70–76
Orthostatic reaction, 65, 71, 81, 87
Osteoarthritis, 54, 65
Osteoporosis, 49, 67–70, 75

P
Package, 105, 108, 123
  leaflet, 105, 108
Partnership, 23, 112, 116, 117
Patient-empowerment, 117
Patient outcome, 21, 31, 33, 95, 121
Personalised medicine, 119, 125, 131
Pharmaceutical care, 95, 115, 119–122, 124, 125, 132
Pharmacodynamics, 3, 9, 14, 15, 39, 103
Pharmacokinetics, 3, 9–14, 17, 39, 79, 103, 108
Pharmacovigilance, 96
Phenotype, 125
Polypharmacy, 1, 2, 4, 9, 49, 65, 67, 71, 74, 75, 98, 108, 111, 113, 122
Practical problems, 101–110, 111, 114, 117, 131
Prescription, 5, 30, 33, 56, 92, 98, 114, 124
Primary care process, 5
Process, 1, 4, 5, 9, 21, 22, 27, 33, 34, 49, 50, 70, 91, 92, 94, 119, 121–126, 129–131
  of aging, 1, 70
  of care, 5, 34, 121
Prostaglandins, 42
Proton pump inhibitors, 54, 56, 57, 103, 106
Psychotic disease, 41, 79, 86

Q
Quality, 1, 2, 4, 21–34, 37, 51–54, 58, 64, 66–68, 71, 73, 75, 76, 84, 102, 119–121, 124, 125, 129, 130
Quality assurance, 21, 23, 120

R
Reflux esophagitis, 56, 57
Registration, 23
Renal failure, 14, 16, 42, 49, 62–64, 72, 75
Research, 22–24, 29, 34, 71, 92, 98, 112, 113, 115, 119, 129, 130
Risks, 1, 4, 21–23, 39, 51, 55, 58, 61, 66, 68, 70, 72, 75, 85, 86, 91, 98, 132
Risperidone, 42, 85

S
Saliva secretion, 52
Sarcopenia, 49, 70, 75
Schizophrenia, 30, 86, 87
Selective serotonin reuptake inhibitor (SSRI), 38, 40, 72, 85, 86, 107
Serum anticholinergic activity, 43
Short product characteristics (SPC), 96, 108
Sleep-wake cycle, 82
Structure, 4, 5, 21, 22, 34, 68, 119, 125, 129–131
Syncope, 14, 17, 71

T
Tardive dyskinesia, 41, 87
To err is human, 33, 93
Trials, 1, 3–5, 22, 25, 26, 28, 30, 59, 96, 102, 108, 131
Tricyclic antidepressants, 16, 43, 50, 72, 82, 85–87
Triggers, 23, 124
Trigger tool, 6, 92, 119, 124, 125

U
Ulcers, 16, 42, 49, 52–56, 58, 75, 94, 105
Urinary incontinence, 49, 55, 58–62, 75, 81, 82

V
Vascular dementia, 84
Vertigo, 49, 65, 73–75

Z
Zolpidem, 40
Zopiclone, 40, 107

GPSR Compliance

The European Union's (EU) General Product Safety Regulation (GPSR) is a set of rules that requires consumer products to be safe and our obligations to ensure this.

If you have any concerns about our products, you can contact us on ProductSafety@springernature.com

In case Publisher is established outside the EU, the EU authorized representative is:

Springer Nature Customer Service Center GmbH
Europaplatz 3
69115 Heidelberg, Germany

Batch number: 10607214

Printed by Printforce, the Netherlands